The American Blood Supply

MIT Press Series in Health and Public Policy
Jeffrey E. Harris, general editor

1. *Professionalism and the Public Interest: Price and Quality in Optometry,* James W. Begun, 1981

2. *Controlling Hospital Costs: The Role of Government Regulation,* Paul L. Joskow, 1981

3. *Biomedical Innovation,* edited by Edward B. Roberts, Robert I. Levy, Stan N. Finkelstein, Jay Moskowitz, and Edward J. Sondik, 1981

4. *An Ounce of Prevention: Child Health Politics under Medicaid,* Anne-Marie Foltz, 1982

5. *The American Blood Supply,* Alvin W. Drake, Stan N. Finkelstein, and Harvey M. Sapolsky, 1982

The American Blood Supply

Alvin W. Drake
Stan N. Finkelstein
Harvey M. Sapolsky

DISCARD

University of Charleston Library
Charleston, WV 25304

The MIT Press
Cambridge, Massachusetts, and London, England

© 1982 by The Massachusetts Institute of Technology

All rights reserved. No part of this book may be reproduced in any form or by any means, electronic or mechanical, including photocopying, recording, or by any information storage and retrieval system, without permission in writing from the publisher.

This book was set in Palatino by Achorn Graphic Services, Inc., and printed and bound by the Murray Printing Co., in the United States of America.

Library of Congress Cataloging in Publication Data

Drake, Alvin W.
  The American blood supply.
  (MIT Press series in health and public policy; 5)
  Includes bibliography and index.
  1. Blood banks—United States. 2. Donation of tissues, organs, etc.—United States. I. Finkelstein, Stan N. II. Sapolsky, Harvey M. III. Title. IV. Series. [DNLM: 1. Blood banks. 2. Blood transfusion. WH 460 D761a]
RM172.D7   362.1'784   82-6599
ISBN 0-262-04070-0   AACR2

Contents

Series Foreword ix

Preface xi-xii

1 The Blood Supply 1
Encounters With the Blood Supply 1
The Blood Supply and its Reputation 4
Donors and Donations 4
The Collection and Distribution of Whole Blood 6
The Pharmaceutical Sector 7
The Uses and the Recipients of Blood 9

2 Ideologies 13
Two Underlying Questions 13
The Four Fundamental Ideologies 15
Ideology and Jurisdiction 18
Ideology and Practice 18
AABB and Red Cross Ideologies 20

3 From Solicitation to Transfusion 22
Recruitment and Collection 22
Processing and Distribution 25
Crossmatching and Transfusion 26
Some Financial Considerations 27

4 Quality 29
Posttransfusion Hepatitis 29
Other Factors in Transfusion and Donation 41
Blood Utilization: The Neglected Area of Quality Control 44
The High Quality of Transfusion Practice 45

5 Nonprofit Organizations 46
The Red Cross Program 47
The American Association of Blood Banks 50
The Failure to Achieve Coordination 54
Strains Within the Organizations 56

6 Profit-Making Organizations: The Plasma Sector 60
The Development of the Plasma Sector 60
Plasma Derivatives and Their Uses 63
The Collection of Plasma 66
The Plasma Business 71
The Future 74

7 Attitudes and Decisions About Donation 76
A Study of Attitudes and Decisions 77
Perceptions of Blood Needs 81
Solicitation and Opportunity to Donate 83
Actual and Perceived Eligibility 85
The Distribution of Donors in the Population 86
Attitudes and Reasons of Nondonors 90
Attitudes and Reasons of Donors 97
Ex-Donors 100
Intense Collection Environments 103
High School Blood Drives 104
The Effects of Ideology and Policy 107
Conclusions 112

8 Cross-National Comparisons 114
The Preference for "Volunteers" 116
Organizational Variations 120
Trading in Blood 121
An Unjaundiced View 124

9 Blood Policy 126
The Underlying Issue 127
The American Blood Commission 130

Controlling Hepatitis   134
The Pharmaceutical Sector   135
Public Participation in the Whole-Blood Supply   137
The Integrity of Public Information   138
Collection Ideology   140
Cartelization and its Consequences   141

Notes   **145**

Index   **159**

Series Foreword

This MIT Press series serves as a forum for significant new research in the field of health and public policy. The series encompasses current problems in health-care organization, financing, and regulation. It also focuses on emerging policy problems in environmental health, workplace safety, toxic substances, and the assessment of new medical technology. We plan to publish original scholarly monographs, highly focused collections by multiple authors, and textbooks that explore new fields.

In this volume, Alvin Drake, Stan Finkelstein, and Harvey Sapolsky of the Massachusetts Institute of Technology provide a comprehensive appraisal of the supply and demand for blood in the United States. The authors—a specialist in operations research, a physician, and a political scientist, respectively—dispel the myth that the American system of blood collection and distribution is inferior to those of other advanced nations. They also clarify the controversy on posttransfusion hepatitis that received so much public and legislative attention a decade ago. They show that many alleged problems in the supply of blood arise from jurisdictional disputes among the major nonprofit blood-banking organizations. They challenge the widespread belief that the American public is reluctant to donate blood. Finally, the authors identify the important issues for blood policy in the United States, such as the consequences of the regionalization of blood services and the need for integrity in blood-collection messages. The book represents a major advance in our understanding of the blood system.

Jeffrey E. Harris

Preface

Although we are all members of the MIT faculty, we came to know each other as a result of our independent interests in blood banking. Al Drake had done operations research on blood-bank inventory control and was involved in a major study of blood-donation attitudes and decisions. Harvey Sapolsky, a political scientist interested in organizations, had prepared a history of the Office of Naval Research, including its contributions to red-cell freezing. Intrigued by the controversy generated by Richard Titmuss's book *The Gift Relationship,* Sapolsky was beginning research on the ways different nations meet their blood needs. Stan Finkelstein, a physician, chemical engineer, and management scientist, was interested in technological innovation in medical care. We began to discuss differences between what "everybody knows" about the blood services complex and the way it appeared to us.

Our book presents an integrated view of many aspects of the blood-services complex. We think the book will be useful to people concerned with technical and administrative aspects of the blood supply. It may also be of interest to people who wish to consider one sector of the health-care delivery system and some of the ways its reputation differs from the facts. We are not concerned here with high technology or biomedical research; these areas of blood banking have a substantial literature. We would like to have been able to deal more explicitly with the economics of blood banking, but the intricacy of that topic led us to believe that the next step in that direction would be a book in itself.

Many individuals have done much to assist us. We have corresponded with and visited more than 100 people, some of whom we returned to several times. The work on donation attitudes and decisions was made possible by grant NIH-5-R01-HS01440 from the National Center for Health Services Research to the MIT Operations Research Center. Comparative studies were sponsored by a grant from the German Marshall Fund. For support on organizational aspects and studies on blood safety we gratefully acknowledge support from the Robert Wood Johnson Foundation and the Commonwealth Fund through the Center for the Analysis of

Health Practices of the Harvard School of Public Health and from the Mellon Foundation through the MIT Program on Science, Technology, and Society.

We owe special gratitude to Geraldine Bourke, Jean Campbell, Cheryl Kelliher, and Judy Spitzer, the capable and patient people who typed and retyped the manuscript as it traveled from author to author to author.

The American Blood Supply

1 The Blood Supply

Encounters with the Blood Supply

Blood, the substance of life, is also the livelihood of thousands of people in the United States. Blood banking is a major health-care enterprise concerned with the collection, processing, distribution, and transfusion of blood and blood products. A network of individuals and institutions known within the trade as the blood-services complex attends to the availability of blood. In the United States, the products and services of this complex are passed on to their eventual users at a total cost in excess of $2 billion each year.[1]

Even when in the best of health, one is never totally divorced from the activities of the blood-services complex. The most common of all encounters with the complex are the inevitable media and personal solicitations for donations. It is unusual for a month to pass during which one does not hear that the quality of medical care in one's community is about to be seriously compromised for want of enough blood donors. General discussions of the blood supply, and much of the publicity associated with particular blood drives, contend that the basic problem is that too few Americans are willing to give their blood.

The inducements to donate vary considerably with the natures of local blood programs. Common incentives include reasons to feel better about oneself, a reduction in hospital charges for a patient one wishes to help, and arrangements known as "blood insurance" or "blood credits" for the donor and for some of the donor's associates. Furthermore, in the yellow pages of telephone directories (under "blood") and in newspaper advertisements one may find opportunities to obtain direct monetary payment.

Most adults know at least one person who has received a blood transfusion. Everyone has a sense that blood is a very special substance, vital to life. Blood-related topics receive an unusual degree of attention, both because of the special considerations the media extend to blood-collection organizations and because of the symbolic nature of blood. The most common topic is the need for blood, either described realistically or dramatized by a blood-program official. The technology of blood science and the development of new medical procedures that involve blood therapy are also taken to be of wide interest. With anticipation, and perhaps a little fear, one reads about developments in the continuing effort to develop "artificial blood."

News and feature stories sometimes appear about particularly questionable arrangements for the collection of blood. We learn about situations in which the facilities, the donors, and the practice of paying donors in cash or in liquor make us concerned about the moral issues and about the risk that we or our loved ones may receive blood products of questionable origin.

Situations experienced by particular patients at the time they need blood can provide topics for news stories. Such cases are used in various ways to document appeals for more blood donations. They also form a basis for discussions of the dependability of the blood supply and of complex issues with regard to equity in blood distribution and in the financial charges associated with blood services. During U.S. Senate Health and Scientific Research Subcommittee hearings in June 1979 on the progress of the National Blood Policy, several dramatic reports were given about the difficulties encountered by particular individuals who needed blood.[2] Although some of these patients had been active donors, they found themselves subject to blood shortages and to apparently excessive charges for the blood they required. Such cases appear in the press somewhat less frequently than they did a few years ago. The distasteful events that form the basis for these stories are sometimes newsworthy, but on occasion the generation of such press items is part of the efforts of two major blood-collection organizations, the American National Red Cross and the American Association of Blood Banks, to embarrass each other.

In the news media or in conversations with friends we may learn about the confusion of patients and their families with regard to the costs associated with blood transfusions. People who have given their blood voluntarily, without any tangible returns, may be surprised at how much they or their insurers are expected to pay for blood products. Similarly, families of patients who have given blood or who have been members of donor groups can be angered when asked to provide additional "replacement blood" or to pay "nonreplacement fees." Couples about to have a child can react with fright and discomfort when asked to join with their friends in "predepositing" blood in case it should be required at the birth.

During the 1979 hearings of the Senate subcommittee on Health and Scientific Research, Senator Richard Schweicker (R, Pennsylvania) attracted considerable attention in the medical and health media by questioning the remarkable variation in the prices charged for identical blood products in different regions of the country. It appeared that the prices of some blood products were based on little more than the whims of local blood-bank administrators.

During the 1970s, television documentaries here and abroad questioned many aspects of the American blood-services complex. Some of them implied broad indictments of our society. Comparisons, light on details but heavy with drama, were made with the ways blood is collected and distributed in other industrialized countries. Furthermore, claims have been made that American pharmaceutical companies purchase the blood of poor people in less developed nations for processing and sale at immense profit.

Two books on the blood supply were published and widely discussed during the 1970s. *The Gift Relationship*, by the eminent British sociologist Richard Titmuss,[3] immediately received much publicity and discussion. Titmuss gave an especially bleak description of the American blood-services complex. He argued, among other things, that the use of money and "blood insurance" as incentives for blood donation made the more altruistic potential donors less likely to participate. This resulted, in Titmuss's view, in a blood supply that was inadequate to meet medical needs and that was also excessively contaminated by hepatitis from paid donors who had good reason to misrepresent their medical histories. In the United Kingdom, Titmuss said, the absence of any tangible payments or rewards for blood inclined a larger fraction of the population to donate. Titmuss believed the underutilization of altruism in the American blood-collection system to be the primary reason for alleged large discrepancies in the quality of blood services in the two countries. His descriptions of the blood supply in the United States were accepted without question by almost all who commented on his work. The book was taken to be a powerful criticism of one aspect of an overly materialistic nation characterized by a lack of commitment to the powerful doctrines of social welfare to which Titmuss ardently subscribed. The other book, *Journey*,[4] told the story of a family determined to yield as little as possible of a son's personal development to his hemophilia. This book also gained wide visibility, including reviews and commentary in national news weeklies and on television discussion programs. Although it may not have been the authors' primary message, many commentators believed the book to show the inadequacy of our arrangements for supplying the blood products hemophiliacs need. The book gave the impression, based on the Massies' experiences in France, that the French had a simpler and more dependable system for supplying blood products to patients with chronic needs.

The Blood Supply and Its Reputation

This book describes significant problems associated with blood policies and practices in the United States. However, our studies lead us to believe that much is right with blood services in this country. We believe that the blood-collection organizations perform far more successfully than would it ever be in their interest to admit. Our research-based conclusions about the willingness of Americans to participate in reasonably well organized blood-collection programs are quite favorable. Comparisons with blood-service practices in some other countries also provide somewhat unexpected results. As one example, we will note that several other advanced nations (whose blood professionals tend to share Titmuss's views of American blood-supply practices) have never solved some of their own blood-supply problems. Some of these countries, in fact, obtain required blood pharmaceuticals from collection and processing facilities located in the United States. An increasing number of such facilities in this country are directly owned by foreign interests.

The issues we will suggest to be of prime importance for the future of the blood supply prove to be quite different from those cited in our opening review of the topics most usually brought to the attention of the public.

Donors and Donations

During 1981 about 8 million people made at least one whole-blood donation in the United States. Although only 5–10 minutes are usually required for the actual drawing of the blood, the donor is typically at the collection site for about 45 minutes. A predonation interview to check on medical status and history, an elementary medical exam, the wait between procedures, and a rest and refreshment period after donation occupy most of the donor's time at the collection site. Having completed a donation of about one pint (actually 450 milliliters, referred to as a unit) of whole blood, the donor is advised to avoid strenuous activity for at least 6 hours and to consume more fluids than usual for the next day or so. With rare exception, blood donors leave a blood-collection location in essentially the same physical condition in which they arrived. The unit of blood taken represents about 10 percent of a typical donor's blood volume. Some components of blood, such as the plasma, will be replaced within the donor's body in a few days. The slowest of the major blood components to regenerate, the red cells, return to their normal level within a few weeks. In the United States, federal regulations require donors to wait at least 8 weeks between whole-blood donations.

The minimum age for blood donation in most states is 17 years. About half the states require parental permission for blood donation by people who are 17 years old. Donors past their mid-sixties may be required to provide recent certification of adequate health from a physician. Other health conditions, recent exposure to several diseases, and medications can make a person temporarily or permanently ineligible for blood donation.

The 8 million or so people who gave whole blood during 1981 averaged about 1.5 donations each, providing a total of about 12 million units of whole blood.[5] The amount collected is determined almost entirely by medical needs, rather than by the willingness of the public to donate or by the capacity of the collection organizations. The number of Americans medically eligible to give blood is much larger than the number of units of whole blood required each year. In fact, our annual whole-blood needs would be more than satisfied if, on the average, every person medically qualified to give whole blood were to make one donation about once every 7 years.

Many whole-blood donors are unclear about what benefits, if any, they receive in turn for their blood. Many do not care. Donors are well aware of the continuing need for blood, and they know there is still no practical substitute for human donors. At present, about a quarter of all whole-blood donations are made, either knowingly or unknowingly, in return for some form of "blood credits" or "blood coverage." There are various forms of such arrangements, all intended to provide blood at reduced cost to donors, their relatives, and their associates. These credit and coverage plans have become less prevalent in recent years. About

70 percent of all whole-blood donations in the United States are now made with no tangible rewards or advantages for the donors. Many donors have the opportunity to give blood at their place of employment during working hours.

A small and declining part of the whole-blood supply, probably on the order of 3–4 percent, is obtained from paid donors.

The Collection and Distribution of Whole Blood

Almost the entire American whole-blood supply is obtained through the collection programs of the American National Red Cross, independent community blood centers, and individual hospitals. In recent years the 57 Red Cross regional blood services collected about half the whole-blood supply,[6] independent community blood centers outside of the Red Cross system collected about 35 percent, and most of the rest was collected by hospitals.[7]

Several modern practices for blood collection, for processing, and for the effective utilization of blood inventories require technologies and administrative procedures that can be impractical for all but the largest individual hospital blood banks. Collecting blood on a planned, predictable basis requires central management of donor recruitment, of mobile collection facilities, and of inventory control and distribution. For these and similar reasons, most individual hospitals have not proved to be effective places for blood collection and processing. There has been a continuing decrease in the fraction of the whole-blood supply drawn in hospitals and a corresponding increase in collections by blood centers.

In the United States, most Red Cross and independent blood centers take responsibility for the collection, processing, and distribution of all or nearly all blood and blood components for most hospitals within their service regions. Many metropolitan areas are serviced by the collection, processing, and distribution capabilities of a single regional blood center. Some metropolitan areas, such as Chicago, are serviced by blood centers (there are several in the Chicago area) and also by significant collection at individual hospitals.

None of the major blood centers now purchase whole-blood donations, although several did until a few years ago. A few hospitals, including some of the most prestigious, meet some of their special needs by purchasing blood from donors. "Professional blood-donor services" and commercial blood-drawing facilities exist in some metropolitan areas. Such firms engage in several activities, one of which is to respond to a hospital's special needs by contacting paid donors and asking them to report to the hospital, sometimes on short notice. Other activities of such firms may be to supply the pharmaceutical sector of the blood supply. It is estimated that in the early 1960s paid donors accounted for as much as a third of the whole blood collected in the United States.[8] At that time, a considerable number of blood centers and hospitals, and a much larger number of commercial collectors than now exist, were paying for at least some of the whole blood they collected.

Depending on the type of chemical preservative used, whole blood (or the red cells separated from it) must be transfused within 3–5 weeks after the blood is drawn; otherwise the blood is said to "outdate." A much more costly procedure, the freezing of red cells, greatly extends the period for which they may be preserved. To hold down outdating, an increasing number of blood centers play an active role in managing the inventory of blood and blood products within their regions. Knowing the status of the blood inventory within an entire region, by type and age, a blood center can redistribute blood as it ages to minimize outdating. Blood centers can also manage the movement of blood from one region of the country to another. Most metropolitan areas are net importers of blood (and hospital patients), using somewhat more blood than they collect. It is common for major metropolitan areas to import 5–25 percent of their blood from collectors in less urban regions. Major blood centers are large enterprises with vehicle fleets, equipment for mobile collection at industrial and community sites, laboratory facilities for testing and processing, storage and distribution facilities, field staffs to promote donor recruitment and organize collection plans, and (especially in the case of Red Cross centers) significant networks to prepare and utilize unpaid volunteers who contribute to blood-drive planning and staffing. Several metropolitan regional blood centers have annual budgets in excess of $20 million.

The Pharmaceutical Sector
Nearly all public experience with and awareness of the blood supply relates to the whole-blood sector. Blood drives and the sup-

porting publicity are concerned almost exclusively with whole blood. However, a "pharmaceutical sector" also has developed. This sector meets medical needs for pharmaceutical products derived from blood plasma.

Red cells and plasma are the two most commonly used components of whole blood. Because they have different therapeutic uses, arrangements must be made to keep the supplies of each in balance with demand. In the United States, as in most other countries that practice modern blood therapy, whole-blood collections are maintained at the level needed to meet medical needs for red cells. The resulting blood collections are not adequate to meet all medical needs for plasma and its derivatives. Very few countries (one of which is Switzerland) collect enough whole blood to meet plasma needs as well as red-cell needs.

Plasma is used for direct transfusion and also as the base for the manufacture of important pharmaceutical products, including albumin (an expensive blood-volume expander that carries minimal risk of disease transmission) and antihemophilic factor (a valuable blood-clotting factor used in significant volume by people with hemophilia). It is the large volume of plasma required for these products that accounts for the fact that, even if all the whole blood collected in the United States were separated into red cells and plasma, the resulting volume of plasma would not be enough to meet the need. Furthermore, meeting all needs for plasma by means of whole-blood collection may be less efficient, and less desirable on medical grounds, than collecting plasma without the red cells that accompany it in whole blood.

The larger part of the need for plasma for pharmaceutical products is attended to by the pharmaceutical sector of the blood-services complex. Most products of this sector are manufactured pharmaceuticals that appear to be prepared best in large quantities using technologies initially developed during World War II.

The pharmaceutical sector obtains most of its plasma by plasmapheresis, a process in which plasma is removed from a portion of the donor's blood and the red cells from that portion are returned to the donor. Because the human body replaces plasma much more rapidly than it replaces red cells, plasmapheresis donors may donate as often as twice a week. Each plasmapheresis donation provides as much plasma as would be obtained from two whole-blood donations. With the technology now available, plasmapheresis donation takes much longer than whole-blood donation. As long as two hours may be required to complete the process of drawing whole blood, removing the plasma, and returning the red cells to the donor's bloodstream.

In the United States, as well as in other countries that draw plasma for the manufacture of pharmaceuticals, far fewer donors participate in the plasma sector than in the whole-blood sector. Some plasmapheresis donors give many times each month. Most plasmapheresis donations in the United States are made to pharmaceutical companies and their agents for direct payments of about $10 or $15. The collection facilities range from major plasma centers (some of which are located near large university campuses) to storefront operations on skid row. Payment for plasmapheresis donations is common practice in most countries that fill their own plasma pharmaceutical needs.

The operations of the pharmaceutical sector of the blood supply are invisible to most Americans. Although exposés about suspicious storefront blood collection sites may not make it clear, they are more often about a pheresis facility than about a whole-blood facility. One obvious area for concern is the possibility that paid plasmapheresis donors, as well as paid whole-blood donors, may have too strong an incentive to misrepresent their state of health. Most plasma-collection facilities in the United States are operated by a small number of pharmaceutical companies and their agents. Many countries have not developed their own plasma supplies. Instead, they purchase plasma that was purchased from donors in the few countries that have, in some form, faced up to the problem of obtaining adequate amounts of plasma from donors.

In the United States, general awareness and most legislative discussion of the blood supply have been concerned only with the whole-blood sector. With the exception of an occasional and possibly sensationalized exposé, the pharmaceutical sector has not been visible enough to stimulate significant public awareness and discussion.

The Uses and the Recipients of Blood

Most prominent blood bankers believe that relatively few medical needs are best served by whole blood. It is increasingly the practice for patients to receive only the particular blood component or components most desirable for their required therapy.[9] This practice, known as component therapy, allows for more efficient utilization of the whole-blood supply and minimizes the recipient's exposure to unneeded substances. The fraction of all transfused units that were in the form of whole blood is estimated to have been more than three times larger in 1971 than it was in 1978.

Whole blood includes red cells, plasma, and platelets, as well as other components used for less common medical procedures. In order to satisfy particular therapeutic needs and to facilitate inventory control, an individual blood component may be made available in several alternative forms. A need for red cells, for example, might be met by transfusing whole blood, or "packed" cells separated out of whole blood, or red cells that have been stored frozen.

Blood serves many vital functions, including transport of nutrients and oxygen, support of the immune systems, and provision of substances for the self-maintenance of the bloodstream (such as clotting proteins). Manufactured pharmaceutical products support some, but not all, blood functions. "Plasma fractions" (substances derived from blood plasma) are required for the manufacture of many of these pharmaceuticals.

Some pharmaceutical products that support blood functions could be made entirely from materials other than human blood. The "artificial blood" fluorocarbons receiving wide attention in the popular press support certain blood functions, particularly oxygen transport. At the time of this writing, no product promises to make a major reduction in the need for human blood donations in the next few years. Several partial substitutes for human blood components and products are and may remain quite expensive in comparison with the human-blood-based materials for which they may be substituted.

The names and functions of the primary components of whole blood are presented in table 1.1. Components such as plasma and platelets, which are rapidly regenerated in the bloodstream of a healthy person, are often obtained by pheresis rather than by separation from donations of whole blood. With the exception of plasmapheresis to provide the needs of the blood-pharmaceutical industry, almost all pheresis donations for individual components such as platelets and white cells in the United States are obtained from unpaid volunteer donors.

Medical procedures requiring blood support may usefully be divided into "elective" procedures (those for which timing is not

Table 1.1 Principal functions of the primary components of whole blood.

	Principal function(s)
Red cells	Oxygen transport
White cells	Defense against infection, breakdown of foreign substances
Platelets	Formation of first clot after tissue injury
Plasma	Maintenance of environment for transport of nutrients and hormones, blood coagulation, immune protection against foreign substances

critical) and "nonelective" procedures (those for which prompt action is of great importance). For the great majority of patients requiring blood transfusion, the immediacy of the medical procedure is not likely to be of major concern. Of course, to ensure the best patient care in all medical procedures, as well as to promote effective utilization of specialized medical facilities and personnel, the blood supply must be very dependable.

The whole-blood supply in the United States is much better than its reputation. Whole blood and blood components are promptly available to the vast majority of patients in need of transfusion. Occasionally, serious availability difficulties do result from catastrophic accidents, from acts of nature, from failures of the collection organizations during holiday periods, and from unusual antibody-typing needs. (Antibodies are circulating substances that support the body's immune systems. For a patient with an especially rare antibody structure it may be difficult to locate compatible blood.)

Many physicians practicing blood therapy have had reason for no more concern about the blood supply than about the water supply.

Only recently—largely through the work of Bruce Friedman—has it become possible to obtain consistent data on transfusion recipients by type of medical diagnosis, by age, and by region of the country.[10] Not surprisingly, a disproportionate fraction of blood transfusions and products go to elderly people, many of whom have chronic diseases. The major classes of diagnoses that result in blood transfusion, and the percentages of the red-cell transfusion volumes they account for, are summarized in table 1.2.

We are aware of no evidence that the whole-blood supply places

Table 1.2 Leading medical diagnoses and conditions resulting in blood transfusions.

	Percentage of all blood transfused
Malignant tumors	18.7
Cardiovascular and cerebrovascular diseases, including open heart surgery	16.1
Accidents	12.0
Blood diseases	5.2
Obstetrical procedures and conditions	4.3
Other diagnoses and conditions[a] accounting for less intensive transfusion	43.7

Adapted from B. A. Friedman, T. L. Burns, and M. A. Schork, A Description and Analysis of Current Blood Transfusion Practices in the U.S. with Applications for the Hospital Transfusion Committee (undated, University of Michigan Medical School and Public Health, Ann Arbor).

a. This large category includes nonmalignant diseases of bones, joints, respiratory tract, gastrointestinal tract, urinary tract, endocrine-reproductive system, musculoskeletal system and skin, vision, hearing, the nervous system; also complications of surgery and medical care, perinatal conditions, nutritional and metabolic disorders, infectious diseases, diabetes mellitus, and hernias.

significant restrictions on the timing or the selection of medical procedures. Very few patients encounter any difficulty due to the availability of blood and blood products. However, some transfused patients may encounter financial or recruitment pressures resulting from their blood needs during hospitalization.

There is usually some exotic new medical procedure under development that appears to require major increases in the nation's blood supply. Although there have been a few periods of more rapid increase, the need for whole blood has not been increasing at an annual rate greater than about 3 or 4 percent in most recent years.[11] The widespread adoption of component therapy during the 1970s contributed to more effective utilization of the whole-blood supply. Better physician education and improved supervision of blood use could also do much to help contain blood needs and allow for better use of the existing supply. We are a long way from running out of willing donors.

2 Ideologies

Ethical questions arise quickly in discussions about the blood supply. Should people who contribute to the blood supply receive preferential treatment when they or their associates need blood? Under what conditions may blood be bought from donors or sold to patients? Is the protection of oneself and one's associates an important incentive for blood donation? If so, is the utilization of this incentive necessary to ensure an adequate blood supply? Are some blood donations, such as pheresis procedures for plasma or platelets, so different from whole-blood donations that ideological views appropriate for whole-blood donations no longer apply?

Two Underlying Questions

The answers to a pair of simple questions are sufficient to specify the fundamental ideology of any blood collection and distribution program.

The first of these questions is "Is it the responsibility of an individual or of society to ensure that blood will be available when the individual needs it?" A response that society is responsible suggests that blood should be thought of as common property and that, when they need blood, donors and their associates should receive no considerations not accorded nondonors. The alternative response suggests that individuals should arrange to provide for their own potential and actual blood needs.

These answers differ sharply with regard to the degree of coupling between a person's participation in the provision of the blood supply and the situation the person may encounter as a patient in need of blood. We call the first ideology *community responsibility* (CR). It requires identical considerations, in every way, for the blood needs of all patients, regardless of whether they or their associates have contributed to the blood supply. The ideology consistent with the second answer we call *individual responsibility* (IR). Individual responsibility allows coupling between a person's participation in the blood supply and some aspect of the situation that arises when that person (or a relative, friend, or co-worker) needs blood.

An individual-responsibility blood program may include features such as requests for the predeposit of blood before admission to a hospital for elective surgery, blood-credit systems of various types, recruitment of family and associates of a patient for blood replacement, recruitment messages promising donors and their associates advantages in time of need, and "nonreplacement fees" for patients who have no provision for replacing (either with blood or with blood credits) the blood they have received. None of these features are allowed under the community-responsibility ideology.

Advocates of each of the two ideologies argue their merits on principle and on the basis of practical consequences. Community-responsibility supporters may insist that all conditions should be identical for all people when they require something as precious and unique as blood. People sympathetic to individual responsibility may insist that it is improper not to offer at least some limited blood-related advantage to the contributors of this precious and unique fluid. At a more practical level, people can debate whether incentives are necessary in order to attract enough donors.[1]

The second underlying question about blood-collection ideology requires less explanation: "May blood be exchanged for money at any point in the collection and distribution system?" We again classify all responses into two groups. One type of response contends that blood should never be exchanged for money or for anything that can be converted into money, that donors should never be paid for their blood and patients should not have to pay for blood. We classify this as the *special gift* (SG) point of view. The alternative point of view contends that blood may be bought and sold, and that a market price reflecting the value of blood may be recognized in monetary as well as in other terms. We refer to this as the *market commodity* (MC) viewpoint.

In practice, people with either point of view accept the notion that blood transfusions will have associated with them charges for costs related to collection, processing, distribution, and transfusion. Admitting only two responses to our second question does present some minor difficulties. There is no entirely satisfactory way to resolve the definition of the phrase "or anything that can be converted into money" that appears in our classification scheme. Most people would agree that coupons for meals at local restaurants or for several gallons of gasoline, however well intended by their sponsors, constitute MC practices. However, there is no clear resolution as to whether allowing blood donors to give blood during working hours is an SG or an MC practice. The tendency is not to consider just enough time off from work to give blood an MC practice.

A collection and distribution system operating under the market-commodity ideology might purchase blood from donors, have a nonreplacement fee, or have a program of blood credit or insurance in which premiums could be paid in money as well as in blood donations. None of these practices is consistent with the special-gift ideology.

The two questions above are adequate for our purpose of discussing a number of ideological structures for blood collection and distribution. One could continue with additional distinctions. For example, in a market-commodity arrangement one could further delineate ideologies according to the two ways blood and money might be exchanged: the purchase of blood from donors and the sale of blood to patients. However, this additional distinction (which may be more important on practical than on ideological grounds, because paying donors may encourage them to misrepresent their health status) will not be needed here.

The four possible combinations of answers to the two questions we have considered—CR-MC, CR-SG, IR-MC, and IR-SG—will serve our purposes of classifying the ideologies of blood collection and distribution systems.

The Four Fundamental Ideologies

Three of the four ideologies are practiced in particular regions of the United States; a fourth (CR-MC) is practiced elsewhere. For clarity, we will outline one example of each of the ideologies. Most of the ideologies are broader than the particular realizations to be given here; the IR-MC ideology includes an especially wide variety of arrangements. To keep the examples brief, we will omit the more obvious assumptions for each example.

CR-MC

As an example of a CR-MC system, consider a national government that purchases blood from citizens who choose to sell it. Suppose also that blood is provided without charge to all patients under a system of nationalized health care.

We designate the system as CR because the treatment afforded patients who need blood is identical in all respects for donors and nondonors. The MC part of the classification follows from the fact that there is an exchange of blood and money (the purchase of blood from donors). If some of the nation's blood supply were purchased and the rest contributed without payment, the system in this example would still be classified as CR-MC. Payment in commodities instead of money would not alter the classification of the example. CR-MC systems for blood collection and distribution are found in Sweden and in a surprising number of socialist and communist countries, including the People's Republic of China.

CR-SG

As an example of the CR-SG ideology, consider a region in which blood donors receive no tangible benefits in return for their donations (which we assume are adequate to meet all needs within the region). Such a region has neither blood-credit systems nor non-replacement fees, and patients needing blood and their associates are subject only to the same donation recruitment effort directed at the general public.

Because no aspect of a patient's situation depends on whether he has participated in some form of contribution to the blood supply, the system is classified as CR. The SG part of the designation results from the absence of any exchange of blood and money. One example of a CR-SG system is the Connecticut Blood Program of the American National Red Cross. Similar programs are to be found elsewhere in the United States, in all of Canada, and in several European countries. The CR-SG ideology, or something very close to it, appears destined to become the dominant blood-collection ideology in the United States.[2]

IR-MC

As one case of an IR-MC system, consider a region in which the blood supply is provided by "donor groups" or "donor clubs"—organizations (such as factories, universities, churches, and social groups) that pay a collective premium in blood donations to cover the potential needs of members and their immediate families. Suppose, as is often the case, that the group members actually provide the region with enough blood to also meet the needs of all or most nonmembers. Nonmembers who receive blood are asked to arrange for replacement, either with blood credits (possibly provided by relatives or friends who are members of donor groups, either locally or elsewhere in the country) or with blood donations. If they are unable to do so, they are charged a nonreplacement fee for each unit of blood received. In effect, these fees subsidize the blood-processing costs for patients who are members of the donor group.

We classify this arrangement as IR because the situation is different for members and nonmembers of the donor groups when they need blood. The MC component of the characterization is due to the fact that, in some circumstances, patients may be required to pay for blood they cannot arrange to replace.

Until recently, the majority of whole-blood collections in the United States were achieved under an IR-MC ideology. In the distant past, when most hospitals had to obtain their own blood supplies without the assistance of regional blood centers and programs, IR-MC systems were almost a necessity in order for individual hospitals to have suitable leverage over an adequate population of potential donors. Several very strong community blood programs continue to operate under IR-MC arrangements. Present examples of this practice include the Irwin Memorial Blood Bank in San Francisco, which fills all blood needs for its geographic region, and the War Memorial Blood Bank in Minneapolis.

IR-SG

As an example of an IR-SG system, consider a region such as the one discussed for IR-MC, in which blood provided by donor groups to cover the needs of their members is adequate to meet most or all of the needs of the entire region. Nonmembers who receive blood are asked to make special efforts to predeposit or replace blood, but the alternative of paying a fee instead of providing blood or blood credits does not exist. Nonmember recipients and their associates are subject to donation requests that are not made to group members when they need blood, and this solicitation is more intense than that experienced by the general public.

Because identical conditions are not presented to all patients at the time they need blood, we designate this system IR. Because it does not allow for a substitution or exchange of blood and money, the system is also designated SG. Many hospital and community blood banks are abandoning their nonreplacement fees while actively recruiting patients and their associates for replacement donations. If it is not already the case, we expect that IR-SG blood collections will soon account for the majority of blood collections in hospital blood banks that do some or all of their own collections. Many urban hospitals, supplied partially or almost completely by central blood programs, augment their blood supplies by active solicitation of relatives and associates of patients.

Ideology and Jurisdiction

Even when the ideology of a particular blood program is clear, there may be difficulty in defining the jurisdiction of the program, which may be in terms of geography or in terms of particular sets of participants. It is easy to think of people who may be subject to, or even caught between, several blood-collection programs with different ideologies. A person who works in Saint Paul (which is almost entirely CR-SG) but who lives in nearby Minneapolis (primarily IR-MC) may be subject to a confusing set of messages and practices. Although the public may have difficulty sorting out conflicting messages about blood ideology, neighboring blood programs generally establish effective and simple procedures for dealing with situations that cross their boundaries without serious consequences for donors or patients.

Ideology and Practice

Although most blood programs have formal ideologies, which are stated most clearly at the highest administrative levels, the practices of a blood program and of the people who assist it are not likely to be entirely consistent with the stated ideology. We will consider here a few examples of the many phenomena that can intervene between ideology and practice, making the practices of different types of blood programs more similar than their ideologies.

We are aware of no present circumstances in which the availability of blood for a patient with immediate needs is in any way related to the patient's blood coverage or financial situation, no matter what the ideology of the local blood collection and distribution system may be. People with immediate needs receive blood in both individual-responsibility and community-responsibility systems. Only in cases of elective medical procedures might an individual-responsibility system differentiate with regard to blood availability between people with and without some form of blood coverage. Even for elective procedures it is extremely unlikely that needed blood products will be denied. Although recruitment messages in individual-responsibility systems may imply more dependable blood availability for donors than for nondonors, it is improbable that this is what happens when blood is actually needed.

People, especially those serving as unpaid volunteer "front line" recruiters for a blood drive at their school, social group, or place of work, tend to deliver recruitment messages with an individual-responsibility flavor, even if the blood program they are assisting is a community-responsibility system. Perhaps a person soliciting blood donations just finds it more fair or expedient to appear to offer people something in return for their blood. This leads to recruitment messages at the personal level that hint, often in a cloudy way, that in time of need some aspect of the situation is better for donors and their loved ones. Similarly, CR-SG blood-collection organizations may try to personalize their blood collections by asking some donors "in whose name" they would like to make their donation—perhaps for some patient the donor knows to have recently received a blood transfusion. In many cases, a CR-SG system will have nothing whatever it can do with this information after it is obtained.

Most mass-media blood messages, whether developed by individual-responsibility or by community-responsibility organizations, deliver essentially the same information to the public. The messages typically remind the public of the continuing need for blood, possibly giving examples of the good use of donated blood and sometimes providing further information about where or how to donate. Mass-media announcements providing individual-responsibility reasons for blood donation are very rare. By implication, mass-media announcements provide community-responsibility reasons for blood donation.[3]

As noted, blood donor groups and clubs in individual-responsibility systems normally provide all or most of the blood supply for the entire population of their region, members and nonmembers. In the increasing number of individual-responsibility systems that have eliminated their nonreplacement fees and lack either the organization or the desire to expose nonmember patients to much additional recruitment pressure, we find blood programs that recruit donors under an individual-responsibility banner but whose practices are actually closer to those of community-responsibility systems.

Because some hospital employees and physicians are very aware of the value of blood and of the perils of an inadequate supply, they may feel compelled to approach patients and their visitors about the importance of replenishing the blood supply. This is one more possible source of individual-responsibility practices in systems intended by their administrators to be of the community-responsibility type.

We have noted five phenomena that make the practices of individual- and community-responsibility blood collection systems less distinct. Severe practical differences between the systems may still exist, particularly from the viewpoint of the family of a patient who has received a considerable amount of blood. But most members of the general public, including many people who are frequent blood donors, are likely to have little concern about, and only a very limited understanding of, the ideology of the blood program in which they participate.

AABB and Red Cross Collection Ideologies

Throughout its history the American Association of Blood Banks has been supportive of blood collection and distribution under IR-MC arrangements. Prior to the development of community blood banks, such arrangements were almost necessary for individual hospitals trying to provide their own independent blood supplies. The IR-MC arrangements also contributed to the structure of the AABB Clearinghouse, an activity that allowed the movement of blood credits among geographic areas. For example, the Clearinghouse made it possible for a family with blood credits in an AABB-affiliated blood bank in New York City to transfer the credits to a relative who needed blood in San Francisco, releasing that relative from the obligation to replace the blood or pay the nonreplacement fee. For many years, the Red Cross also participated in the activity of the AABB Clearinghouse.

Although AABB-member blood banks are free to choose their own collection ideologies, the AABB and almost all its members have argued for the desirability of IR-MC systems. The avoidance of future nonreplacement fees was claimed to provide a major incentive for blood donors, most of whom were judged to be more likely to want to protect themselves and their families than to be willing to give their blood to the community at large. Furthermore, one can claim to find justice in either system. In principle, requiring patients without blood credits to replace blood is merely asking these people to contribute to the replenishment of the blood supply, as patients with blood credits have already done.

Different financial arrangements developed in AABB and Red Cross blood programs. Under the AABB programs, about half the patients without blood coverage paid nonreplacement fees rather than provide replacement blood. This came to be an important aspect of the fiscal structure of most AABB blood banks.

In many regions of the country, including several in which it was an active blood collector, the Red Cross's positions with regard to blood-collection ideology were, for a long period of time, of almost no consequence to anybody. As recently as 1970 or so, many Red Cross Centers were unable to come close to meeting most needs of the hospitals in their regions. As long as this situation prevailed, the Red Cross could not dictate many of the arrangements under which hospitals were to use Red Cross blood. In fact, although the Red Cross did not support the concept of nonreplacement fees, it did attempt to maintain its own blood-credit system. Some hospitals required that each unit of blood be replaced by several units in order to eliminate the nonreplacement fee. The Red Cross might have no alternative to cover the needs of its donors other than to go along with this practice. Like some of the other IR-MC practices, the multiple-replacement notion had more validity years ago when most hospitals had to generate their own blood supplies (which generally could not be done with the efficiencies and utilization rates possible in larger systems). In recent years, the Red Cross has moved to a strong position endorsing the community-responsibility ideology.

3 From Solicitation to Transfusion

Whole-blood collections in the United States have grown from about 1–2 million units in 1950 to about 12 million units in 1981.[1] Today, a region that meets its own blood needs requires about one unit of whole blood per year for about every 20 people in the region. The mobilization of the resources needed to meet the growing blood supply and the higher technology of the system has resulted in increased specialization and professionalization at all stages of the process, from the solicitation of potential donors to the transfusion. Major steps in this chain include the solicitation of donors, the planning and execution of collections, and the processing, distribution, crossmatching, and transfusion of the blood.

As blood banking became a common practice for civilian health care in the United States during and after World War II, it was commonly the case that all of these steps were performed within individual hospitals under IR-MC arrangements.[2] A few regions of the country were served by dependable centralized blood centers as early as 1950. Most major hospitals, however, found it necessary to raise all or part of their own whole-blood supplies, sometimes assisted by central blood programs (which were often not capable of total supply) and also assisted in many parts of the country by commercial firms that purchased blood from donors.

Each step of the blood-banking process requires a different mix of professional skills and regional coordination. Most of the steps also involve issues of organizational visibility, autonomy, accountability, and revenue. With the exception of crossmatching and transfusion, the major steps have generally been moving out of hospitals and becoming functions of other organizations.

Recruitment and Collection

Efforts of many types can precondition a broad population to make it more receptive to solicitation for blood donation. Few of these efforts can be performed well by an individual hospital, with some exceptions for a hospital that is unusually large or is the only blood collector in its region. The experience in regions where several hospitals or blood centers compete for the same donor population has been especially poor in terms of efficiency and coordination of the blood supply. Houston in 1975 and Chicago today are examples of areas in which too many collectors and too little coordination have resulted in inefficient and sometimes inadequate voluntary whole-blood supplies.[3]

Educational programs about blood and blood needs, including consistent press and media relations, are services most effectively provided by regional blood centers, which are able to speak to many listeners with a single voice. Further support comes at the national level. Major public education programs prepared by organizations such as the American Association of Blood Banks and the American National Red Cross are given directly to the media and to regional and local blood programs for further dissemination. Public education programs, usually sets of brief messages with a consistent theme, may be prepared and propagated with the cooperation of media organizations, especially the National Advertising Council.

Nobody doubts that a continuing public awareness of blood needs is conducive to blood collection. Some of our research suggests that the level of this preconditioning may already be adequate. It does not appear necessary to provide much more public education with regard to blood needs and the wonders of blood processing and utilization in order to achieve an adequate response to well-organized collection programs.

Whether or not it is desirable to offer donors tangible benefits in return for their blood is both an ideological and a practical issue. Although the ideological question remains forever open to personal choice, we believe the practical question has been resolved. A number of blood programs in the United States and abroad provide firm demonstrations that offers of donation benefits are not necessary to sustain a community's blood supply. The regional blood programs in Connecticut and in upstate New York have long been able to meet local needs without offering any individual-responsibility incentives.

There was a period when the messages from most blood collectors, whether they were individual hospitals or Red Cross or independent blood centers, were of the "give blood to protect yourself and those dear to you" sort. Particularly in the written materials for the "blood protection plans" offered to potential donors, one found hints that blood availability was somehow much better for participants than for nonparticipants. The incentive of release from nonreplacement fees was also promoted by most blood-collection programs. These still are among the messages from blood collectors committed to IR-MC ideology and practices. Partly because of the large volunteer component in the staffing and execution of large collection efforts, especially those of the Red Cross, it is remarkable to note how many of the old IR-MC messages still are perpetuated in blood-collection systems that now describe themselves as CR-SG. Red Cross volunteers and even some Red Cross professionals are still delivering recruitment messages that the organization believes it abandoned many years ago.

Blood-donation solicitation, in a variety of forms, reaches most Americans surprisingly often. The forms range from the most general public information to personal requests, including the now less common solicitation to help replace blood for a friend in an individual-responsibility system. Donor-solicitation efforts also include actual and sometimes staged "blood crisis" campaigns, usually leading to the appearance of too many donors in too short a time for the collecting agency to make the best use of their blood.

The majority of American adults already believe they have regular, convenient opportunities for blood donation. It may well be that the vital part of donor recruitment for modern blood practice is simply the provision of convenient, realistic donation opportunities, coupled with personal recruitment chains to reach an adequate number of potential donors. Regional planning and scheduling of donation opportunities are far more worthwhile than is exhorting the general public to give blood at unspecified times and places.

There has been a nationwide trend for blood collections to be made at places where there are significant numbers of potential donors—especially workplaces. The development and maintenance of the necessary mobile collection facilities require, in addition to experienced personnel and the willingness of employers to sacrifice employee time, a large enough region of operation to allow the best use of the specialized equipment and personnel required. Equipment and personnel scheduling typically is required several months in advance. Potential collection sites have proved more receptive to a visit request from a region's central blood-collection organization than to competitive requests from several collection organizations within a region.

Coordination of a region's blood-collection activities also has made possible consistency in the solicitation messages reaching the public. For a potential donor or collection site to have to compare the benefits of affiliation with alternative collection organizations may, in the long run, provide unneeded impediments to blood donations for which such considerations are likely to be of little consequence or relevance. Of course, new difficulties may arise when a monopoly on blood collection and distribution is given to a single organization.

Processing and Distribution

Effective processing of collected whole blood is beyond the reach of all but the largest individual hospital blood banks.

After being typed and tested for potential disease transmission (including hepatitis, for which the best existing tests are quite inadequate), most of the donated whole blood is broken down into its components. Each component requires storage under appropriate conditions and careful management of the resulting inventory to minimize outdating.

Depending on the chemical preservative used, the shelf life of whole blood or the red cells separated from it is regulated to be either 3 or 5 weeks. Blood banks are faced with the management of large quantities of a perishable, type-specific inventory. There is a significant literature on the management of blood inventories.[4] Good management, providing a low average age of blood at the time of transfusion while balancing the resulting outdating and shortage rates, requires a sophisticated information and needs-projection system. In many cases, these capacities are complemented by transportation systems with the capacity to redistribute blood among hospitals and to return blood from hospitals to a central inventory at a regional blood center.

Such arrangements for the management of a region's blood supply require that the hospital blood banks allot certain management powers to a single regional organization. Hospitals—the places where blood is transfused—have historically been hesitant to leave inventory-control decisions in the hands of a body that could not ensure a dependable supply of blood products when they might actually be required at the hospitals. In earlier years, for example, many hospitals relinquished their own collection programs and control over their inventories to Red Cross blood centers that, in the long or the short run, proved unable to meet hospital needs for blood and blood products.[5]

Central tracking and utilization of a region's blood resources do not require that there be a single collection agency in the region. There is, however, an intimate coupling between the planning and execution of blood collections and the management of blood inventories, including possibilities for their redistribution. More local and less formal systems of inventory swapping and sharing tend to result in less effective inventory utilization than that which is at least theoretically achievable by totally centralized inventory management.

Crossmatching and Transfusion

After the possible blood needs of a hospital patient awaiting a medical procedure have been estimated, blood of the appropriate type will be, in all but the most urgent cases, crossmatched to ensure that it is compatible with the patient's antibody structure. For the great majority of blood uses that are elective, as well as in some emergency cases, blood crossmatched to a particular patient is placed on reserve in the hospital blood bank until the medical procedures are performed. Because prudent planning requires the reservation of more blood than patients will use, some larger hospital blood banks may have some units of blood simultaneously on reserve for any of several potential users.

Very specialized crossmatching requirements, although unusual, can require extensive data bases and information systems to locate, either in blood-bank inventories or in willing potential donors on "rare donor" lists, blood of the appropriate type and antibody structure. In emergencies where immediacy of need is an overwhelming factor, less satisfactory crossmatches (or none at all) may be acceptable to balance the timing of the needed transfusion with the risk of complications due to a mismatch.

Except for a very few regional blood banks that are supported by outstandingly effective blood-transportation services,[6] crossmatching is performed within hospital blood banks, which in special cases may require outside assistance to find compatible blood. Although many steps intercede between donor and patient, the overwhelming majority of hospital patients receive the blood therapy they need without undue delay.

Some hospitals say they have active review committees to

monitor the effectiveness with which they utilize blood. Unless the hospital blood-bank director has and wields sufficient authority, all physicians (many of whom are not too aware of modern blood therapy practices) are likely to get whatever they request from the hospital blood bank. Some people suspect that the weakest link in the blood supply is often the misutilization resulting from ineffective transfusion practices.[7]

Some Financial Considerations

The billing for blood and blood services, either to the patient or to his insurers, is carried out by the hospital blood bank through the hospital's financial office. In individual-responsibility hospital blood banks, the eventual resolution of the bill may require communication with one or more blood-collection organizations outside the hospital.

Costs of many kinds are associated with provision of blood. By the time the patient is billed, costs have been incurred for public donation education and for collection and processing. Some other, less visible costs will be paid by other parties.

General public education about blood needs and blood donation does not provide visible short-term benefits for most parties in the blood-services complex. All participating organizations eagerly encourage other participants to develop and to pay for public education campaigns. The national blood-collection organizations, supported by the good will of the media, do a significant amount of work in this direction. There is some controversy about the payoff of and need for extending such efforts. Public education programs also provide increased public visibility for organizations such as the Red Cross that have additional reasons to keep the public aware of the services they provide.

The planning and execution of blood collections to provide a relatively uniform blood supply on a consistent basis, especially through mobile operations, is an extensive and expensive operation. As a striking example of some of the hidden costs, professional donor recruiters have estimated that mobile blood collections at an industrial site, especially those where workers leave assembly lines in order to donate blood, can easily cost the employer $50 or more per unit of blood collected. This includes not only the direct disruption of production, but also the many other supporting services provided by the employer before and during the collection visit. Such expenses may be included in the employer's product prices, but they do not appear in the expenses of the blood-collection organization. (Because paid donors require little additional solicitation and deliver themselves to fixed, less expensive collection facilities, one can see merit in the argument made by commercial blood collectors that paying for whole blood may be the least expensive way to obtain it.) Direct recruitment and collection costs are passed on, along with laboratory and other costs, as part of the "processing fee" the patient will be billed along with an "administration fee" (covering expenses of the transfusion itself) for blood products used.

This is not a book on blood-bank economics, a field fraught with the complexities of multiple products produced from a single source by a variety of public and private organizations. However, it is clear that simple blood-policy decisions may have major financial implications for all concerned. Even within an individual hospital blood bank, decisions about crossmatch policy (How much blood should be crossmatched and placed on reserve for a procedure scheduled for a particular patient? For how many patients may a unit of blood be crossmatched and reserved at any one time?) have major impacts on revenues and the allocation of charges. It is our impression that blood banks have been among the financially rewarding areas of hospital activity.

Although it is less of an issue as the practice diminishes, many hospital blood banks have improved their financial positions by considerably inflating the nonreplacement fee. A hospital or a blood center that asks a patient to pay for blood used with money or with blood donations is most likely hoping to have the payment made in money rather than in blood.

4 Quality

As the evolving science and practice of blood transfusion has facilitated major advances in the treatment of disease, it has become an indispensable part of clinical medicine. Blood transfusion is relatively safe, but not risk-free. Considerable effort is expended by trained personnel to ensure that the processes of blood collection and transfusion are conducted in a manner that preserves the quality of the transfusion product and minimizes the risk of compromise to recipient and donor.

Posttransfusion Hepatitis

Posttransfusion hepatitis has been the most visible quality issue and a centerpiece of the public-policy debate over blood banking. Hepatitis, or inflammatory liver disease, encompasses a number of different disorders whose origins include viruses, alcoholic excess, and medical therapies. The chief symptoms are likely to be similar, irrespective of the cause: yellowing of the skin and possibly incapacitating malaise lasting for a period of weeks to months. Laboratory tests are capable of establishing the cause of a relatively small proportion of the cases. The medical history of the patient often proves more useful in determining the source of the disease. Prevention of hepatitis by a vaccine is possible in some instances; however, there is no cure. In a typical year, about 50,000 cases are reported to public health officials[1] and some believe as many as 150,000 more are not reported. Deaths from hepatitis are rare (about 1–3 percent of all cases[2]) and generally limited to the elderly and others suffering from chronic diseases.

Most cases of hepatitis result from infection with one of three classes of viruses, referred to as type A, type B, or type non-A, non-B.[3] Length of incubation period can be informative for distinguishing among cases caused by the different viruses. Hepatitis A has a short incubation period (30–45 days), seasonal variation, and is associated with shellfish, epidemics, and natural disasters but practically never with transfusion. Preschool and school-age children are frequent victims. Type B has a longer incubation period (90–180 days) and tends to afflict an older group. For the non-A, non-B variety, the incubation period is thought to be intermediate, possibly even as short as that of type A. The B and non-A, non-B viruses are the most frequent causative agents of hepatitis in blood recipients. Studies have shown that the clinical severity of the disease and the fatality rate are more closely related to the age of the patient than to the virus type, with younger patients suffering lower morbidity and mortality.[4]

Generally effective laboratory screening is possible for type B hepatitis. Blumberg discovered in 1964 that a virus-derived serum particle, later named the "hepatitis B surface antigen" (HBsAg), is identifiable in the blood of individuals carrying type B disease.[5] This Nobel Prize–winning discovery was the basis for the highly sensitive screening tests for hepatitis B now used routinely in blood banks.[6] A vaccine against hepatitis B currently in clinical testing was also a product of this line of research;[7] after it becomes generally available it should prove useful in protecting high-risk population groups.

Until recently, type B virus was thought to be the most important determinant of posttransfusion hepatitis. However, although the introduction into common use of the latest generation of screening tests based on the hepatitis B surface antigen virtually eliminated virus type B as a complication of transfusion, many cases of hepatitis still occurred.[8] In several institutional research settings it became possible to confirm the presence of the non-A, non-B viral causative agents for nearly all of the remaining transfusion-hepatitis cases.[9] Unfortunately, progress toward identifying the non-A, non-B virus has been slow. Partially effective screening for non-A, non-B hepatitis may be accomplished by testing the level of the enzyme alanine aminotransferase in the donor's blood.[10]

Between 3 and 10 percent of blood recipients may develop hepatitis. As many as 120,000 cases may occur each year in the United States.[11] Between 0.4 and 6.0 of each 1,000 units of blood transfused may be infected with hepatitis virus.[12] Table 4.1 summarizes the range of projected occurrence rates.

The exact magnitude of the risk and the patient's chances of becoming seriously ill with hepatitis have historically been difficult to estimate. Contributing to the overstatement of the risk is the fact that transfusion is only one of a number of causes of hepatitis in blood recipients. Anyone showing signs of inflammatory liver disease within a year of a transfusion might be

Table 4.1 Incidence of posttransfusion hepatitis.

	Lowest estimate	Highest estimate
Cases/Year[a]	92,000	120,000
Deaths/Year[a]	1,000	3,700
Risk (cases/1,000 units transfused)	0.4[b]	6[c]

a. Source: ref. 11.
b. Source: Taswell et al., ref. 12.
c. Source: Seeff et al., ref. 12.

counted in the transfusion-hepatitis category with some justification. Contributing to the understatement of the risk is the observation that the disease remains undiagnosed and hence unreported much of the time.[13]

Keeping track of the occurrence rates of posttransfusion hepatitis is a responsibility of the federal Center for Disease Control (CDC) and of the state Public Health Departments, which report actual case incidences to the CDC. This reporting channel has been only partly effective. The number of cases specifically identified as posttransfusion hepatitis and reported to the CDC is very low; others have been aggregated into larger categories such as "serum hepatitis" or remain unreported. The CDC supplements its case reports with data collected from special hepatitis surveys to attempt to define the extent of the posttransfusion hepatitis problem (note 2). The CDC estimated that there were 92,000 cases in 1970 (note 11). This number is short of the 120,000 cases some believe occur per year.

Alternatively, data from clinical research studies can be used to project the percentage of all hepatitis cases that were transfusion-related. One approach would be to aggregate data reported by hospitals and clinics treating posttransfusion hepatitis patients. In eleven studies carried out between 1946 and 1965 and reviewed in 1973, the mean attack rate was 4.1 cases of hepatitis per 1,000 units of blood transfused.[14] Multiplying this rate by 6.4 million, the number of units transfused in 1971, accounts for about 26,000 cases of posttransfusion hepatitis. This estimate is consistent with the findings of the National Transfusion Hepatitis Study, a cooperative study of 14 university medical centers that reported in 1972 about 20,000 overt cases of posttransfusion hepatitis.[15] However, both of these projections are considerably lower than the 92,000 cases the CDC believes occur annually.

Much of the difference may be due to variations in the intensity of patient followup. A minority of institutions actively solicit status information from transfusion recipients at regular intervals. Many do little to follow up transfusion other than wait for case reports to arrive through the mail from attending physicians. There are few incentives for the practitioner to complete such reports, and a hospital may fail to acknowledge hepatitis cases to preserve its reputation. A ten-year study by the New Jersey State Department of Health[16] found that, on the average, 30 percent of the posttransfusion hepatitis cases that were eventually identified by intensive record review had originally been missed. Occasionally, research studies are designed and conducted to carefully follow a sample of transfusion recipients for the development of hepatitis.

Other research studies have been concerned with the frequency of occurrence of hepatitis B surface antigen in the donor population as determined by blood-bank screening tests.[16,17] Hepatitis B may currently be the cause of about 5–25 percent of transfusion-related cases; the remainder may be the result of infection with the non-A, non-B virus.[18] The prevalence of HBsAg in the population should be proportional to the threat of the type B variety of the disease.

Reliable projections of mortality rates from posttransfusion hepatitis have proved even more difficult than case occurrence rates. Estimates ranging from 1,000 to 3,700 deaths per year have been reported in the literature (note 11).

Whatever the magnitude of the posttransfusion-hepatitis problem, there has been interest in identifying blood-collection practices that are associated with high hepatitis risk. Much interest has centered on the characteristics of donor populations having a high likelihood of transmitting disease. In the absence of laboratory screening tests for the prevention of posttransfusion hepatitis that could routinely detect the presence of non-A, non-B virus, studies of the demographic and social variables that might discriminate between high and low likelihood of transmitting or receiving posttransfusion hepatitis may have practical implications. For example, it has been widely suggested that payment for blood increases the frequency of posttransfusion hepatitis.

Much has been written about the characteristics of blood donors that influence their likelihood of transmitting hepatitis. We now review and discuss a number of these possible relationships.

Paid-for commercial blood is associated with a higher hepatitis risk than blood not paid for.

Numerous studies have addressed the relationship between whole blood collected by profit-making blood banks and the attendant risks of hepatitis from a transfusion. Nearly all have concluded that commercial blood is riskier. The magnitude of the difference in risk varied considerably from one study to the next.

Hepatitis-occurrence data from two Veterans Administration hospitals in Boston between 1952 and 1957 offered qualitative evidence of the association between hepatitis risk and commercial donors.[19] A higher-than-expected incidence of hepatitis was noted in certain years when a large fraction of the whole blood transfused at one of the hospitals was purchased from a single commercial source.

In 1970, J. Garrott Allen published data collected many years earlier (1946–1957), encompassing over 56,000 blood donations. He concluded that a unit of commercially obtained whole blood then carried 10–25 times the hepatitis risk of a unit given by an unpaid donor.[20] The National Transfusion Hepatitis Study also addressed this question and reported on it in 1972. On the basis of data on nearly 5,000 cardiovascular-surgery patients who had received an average of almost 8 units of blood each, 3–6 times the risk of posttransfusion hepatitis was noted with paid over unpaid blood (note 15). For cardiac-surgery patients treated at the National Institutes of Health, researchers estimated that the elimination of commercial blood transfusions could lead to as much as a 70 percent drop in posttransfusion hepatitis.[21] Hospital record studies conducted by the New Jersey Department of Public Health, covering the period 1967–1976, demonstrated a 4–10-times-greater risk of posttransfusion hepatitis with commercial blood.[22] During the period of the New Jersey study, the risk of acquiring hepatitis after a blood transfusion declined from almost one in 500 to nearly one in 3,000. (A small portion of this decline probably can be attributed to the increasing use of the laboratory screening tests for hepatitis B that were introduced during this period.)

Some un-paid-for blood may have a higher risk of transmitting hepatitis than some paid-for blood.

All un-paid-for blood is not necessarily superior to all paid-for blood, in part because not all paid-for blood is commercial. Nonprofit hospitals and blood banks that pay some donors may do so without adversely affecting hepatitis transmission rates. In the early 1970s, the U.S. General Accounting Office (GAO) sought to test the popular conception that a patient receiving a blood transfusion had a higher risk of developing hepatitis if the donor had been paid (ref. 11). Table 4.2 lists 14 geographically distributed blood-collection centers along with GAO data on posttransfusion hepatitis. The Houston center, using 100 percent paid-for blood, had a more favorable hepatitis case rate than three other centers: Boston and Columbus, both of which used no paid-for blood, and Denver, which used less than 1 percent paid-for blood. On the basis of data from 39 blood banks in 4 cities, the GAO concluded that certain paid donors were less likely to transmit hepatitis than certain volunteer donors. In table 4.3, the prevalence of hepatitis B antigen per 1,000 units of blood screened is presented as a function of whether or not donors were paid. The 10 blood banks with

Table 4.2 Incidence of posttransfusion hepatitis according to percentage of commercial blood and geographic location.

Location of medical center	Cases per 100 patients	Percentage of paid commercial blood
Lexington, Ky.	—	3
Rochester, Minn.	0.5	<1
Minneapolis, Minn.	0.6	<1
Atlanta, Ga.	2.0	—
San Francisco, Calif.	2.1	—
Houston, Tex.	2.2	100
Baltimore, Md.	2.3	24
Boston, Mass.	2.3	—
Indianapolis, Ind.	2.6	36
Columbus, Ohio	3.1	—
Cleveland, Ohio	3.3	44
Denver, Colo.	4.7	<1
Chicago, Ill.	8.1	38
Los Angeles, Calif.	8.6	57
Overall average	2.8	21

Source: ref. 11.

Table 4.3 Hepatitis B antigen positivity rates of 39 nonprofit blood banks.

Donor group	Paid or volunteer[a]	Rate per 1,000	Donor group	Paid or volunteer[a]	Rate per 1,000
A	V	—	T	V	2.0
B	V	—	U	P	2.1
C	P	—	V	P	2.2
D	V	0.6	W	V	2.8
E	V	0.8	X	V	2.9
F	P	0.8	Y	P	3.0
G	P	0.8	Z	P	3.5
H	V	0.9	AA	V	3.8
I	V	1.0	BB	V	4.1
J	P	1.3	CC	P	4.3
K	V	1.3	DD	P	4.4
L	V	1.3	EE	P	4.4
M	V	1.3	FF	V	4.7
N	V	1.4	GG	P	4.8
O	V	1.4	HH	P	5.0
P	V	1.5	II	V	5.6
Q	V	1.5	JJ	P	6.7
R	V	1.8	KK	P	6.8
S	V	1.8	LL	P	9.0
			MM	P	11.0

Source: ref. 11.
a. V indicates all donors unpaid; P indicates some donors paid.

the most favorable hepatitis B prevalence rates included 4 centers that paid certain well-defined and carefully controlled populations of donors. The 10 blood banks with the least favorable hepatitis B antigen rates included 2 centers that used only volunteers. At least three other studies address this issue. In 1971, the Massachusetts Department of Public Health examined records of 85,000 units of blood and found hepatitis B antigen positivity only 60 percent as great in blood banks using some paid donors as in those that only take blood from volunteers (Massachusetts Department of Public Health, ref. 17). Similar findings were reported in 1973 at the U.S. Army Fitzsimmons Medical Center that found the hepatitis B antigen prevalence in a study of 6,000 units to be only 10 percent as great among its paid donors as among its volunteers (Holley and Linkenhofer, ref. 17). Blood Services, Inc., a chain that operated more than 20 blood banks in 14 southern and western states, changed its blood-collection practices during 1972–1973. Blood Services converted gradually over that two-year period from a donor-payment incentive program to a 100 percent unpaid community-responsibility system. The increasing use of unpaid donors was associated with an increasing case incidence of posttransfusion hepatitis.[23] However, part of this increase may be attributable to improved hepatitis case reporting.

Unfavorable socioeconomic conditions of blood donors correlate with greater risk of posttransfusion hepatitis.

In an effort to correlate hepatitis risk with socioeconomic conditions, GAO auditors asked blood-bank officials for the precise geographical areas from which their donors were drawn (ref. 11). The GAO selected 21 donor populations for which the hepatitis B antigen screening techniques in use were approximately the same. A socioeconomic profile of the "catchment areas" for the donor populations, including income and housing characteristics, was developed from 1970 census data. As table 4.4 shows, the mean hepatitis B antigen positivity rate was about 1.5 per thousand units screened for the unpaid donor groups and more than 3 times greater for the paid donor groups. But socioeconomic characteristics of the donors were more strongly correlated to the hepatitis antigen B positivity rate than to whether the donors were paid or unpaid. Socioeconomic factors explained 63 percent of the differences between the hepatitis antigen rates in the various donor populations, whereas payment explained only 36 percent.

Table 4.4 Hepatitis B antigen frequency rates and socioeconomic characteristics of donor populations of 19 blood banks.

Donor groups	Paid or volunteer	HBsAg positives per 1,000	Income characteristics		Housing characteristics		
			Percentage below poverty level	Estimated median family income	Percentage lacking complete plumbing	Percentage lacking complete kitchen	Percentage built before 1940
A	V	0.0	10.9	$ 4,371	1.2	1.1	18.0
D	V	0.6	5.6	11,915	0.6	1.0	7.5
E	V	0.8	11.9	7,730	8.1	5.9	79.1
F	P	0.8	4.8	7,745	2.2	0.5	10.5
H	V	0.9	3.9	11,075	1.5	0.5	22.3
K	V	1.3	2.8	13,831	1.1	0.8	17.9
L	V	1.3	2.8	13,831	1.1	0.8	17.9
N	P	1.4	8.2	10,282	1.5	1.6	31.6
O	V	1.4	8.2	10,282	1.5	1.6	31.6
X	V	2.9	2.2	13,627	1.7	0.7	13.5
Y	P	3.0	13.0	7,542	2.2	2.6	47.6
Z	P	3.5	9.9	10,535	1.9	3.2	32.2
CC	P	4.3	11.9	7,730	8.1	5.9	79.1
DD	P	4.4	15.4	8,642	5.0	3.2	66.1
EE	P	4.4	13.8	8,676	2.3	1.3	68.0
FF	V	4.7	26.2	6,843	3.2	3.7	82.4
HH	P	5.0	20.6	7,500	2.8	3.3	79.3
KK	P	6.8	13.0	7,542	2.2	2.6	47.6
LL	P	9.0	17.5	8,251	6.5	5.3	75.5

Source: ref. 11

Socioeconomic characteristics of blood donors were also studied by researchers at the New Jersey Department of Health (ref. 22). They assembled hepatitis B antigen positivity rates for unpaid donations during 1970 in four New Jersey counties which differed widely in terms of the socioeconomic composition of their inhabitants. Rates were highest in the areas with the least favorable housing facilities and family incomes.

Age, sex, race, and previous blood donation can be predictors of the risk of posttransfusion hepatitis.

A 1972–1973 study by the Greater New York Blood Program of 128,000 unpaid blood donors concluded that age, sex, race, religion, and level of education correlated with hepatitis B antigen positivity in their study sample.[24] Donors less than 20 years of age and over 50 (a very small portion of the donor pool at that time) were disproportionately less frequent carriers of hepatitis antigen than donors between the ages of 20 and 49. Women were less frequent carriers of hepatitis B than men. Hepatitis B antigen was detected five times as frequently among non-Caucasian as among Caucasian donors. Jews were found to be hepatitis B antigen positive less frequently than Catholics and Protestants. Higher educational level correlated with lower hepatitis-antigen prevalence.

The strongest correlation found by the New York researchers was the nearly 10 times as frequent hepatitis B antigen positivity among first-time donors as among repeat donors (table 4.5). Donors who have given blood in the past without being implicated in a case of hepatitis seem to be, from a hepatitis-transmission standpoint, the safest donors that can be found (ref. 24).

Table 4.5 Frequency of hepatitis B antigen in first-time and repeat donors.

	No. of hepatitis B antigen positives/ No. of units screened	Hepatitis B antigen prevalence per 1,000 units of blood collected[a]
First-time donors	126/67,092	1.90
Repeat donors	13/61,141	0.21

Source: ref. 24.
a. Standardized for sex and age.

(A positive HBsAg test is, of course, grounds for future deferral of that donor.)

Posttransfusion hepatitis has declined over time.

Decreasing use of commercial blood and increasing acceptance of hepatitis B antigen screening tests must have contributed to declining incidence and death rates from posttransfusion hepatitis. Many experts believe that the increased reliance on unpaid donors is the most significant factor contributing to the continuation of the trend toward declining rates of posttransfusion hepatitis. The decline in death rates alone from hepatitis B may have been as much as fivefold (ref. 8). As stated, hepatitis B virus is a much less frequent cause of the disease than the non-A, non-B agents (ref. 18). Recently, researchers have reported some hope of reducing non-A, non-B hepatitis by screening donors' blood for abnormal levels of the enzyme alanine aminotransferase (ALT). There are many unanswered questions about the efficacy of ALT for this purpose.[25] The ALT screening test is neither very sensitive nor specific, and, if fully implemented, could result in the deferral of many healthy donors.[26]

The risk of hepatitis differs from whole-blood to component transfusion.

Much of the data presented above relates specifically to the risks of contracting hepatitis associated with the transfusion of whole blood. The risk may be different for some blood components and products. Several studies suggest an improvement in hepatitis risk with the transfusion of frozen and washed red cells.[27] Freezing red cells requires the introduction and later removal of glycerol to protect the cells from damage during the freezing and thawing stages. Before transfusion, the glycerol is removed by an extensive washing process. The resulting product may be safer than the original blood from which it came. Recent research has not fully supported the claim of reduced hepatitis risk of frozen red cells.[28] In theory, it is also possible that institutions able to make a capital investment in the blood-freezing technology may also be those that attract and maintain a higher-quality pool of donors and hence less hepatitis-contaminated blood.

Hepatitis risk is known to be less with transfusions of certain processed blood derivatives. The plasma protein albumin has been studied extensively for hepatitis risk. Data suggesting that albumin is free of hepatitis risk has been interpreted to be a favorable result of the heat-treatment process, sometimes called pasteurization, that is performed during its manufacture.[29] Other plasma derivatives, such as the antihemophilic proteins and concentrates, are apparently associated with a substantial risk of hepatitis transmission when transfused. However many of the surviving recipients of the antihemophilic proteins receive transfusions frequently and as many as 90 percent have developed circulating immunity to hepatitis B virus. This observation could explain the relatively low incidence of hepatitis-B among hemophiliacs. An increasing number of hemophiliacs, however, seem to be contracting acute non-A, non-B hepatitis.

For many years, public interest has been aroused by the problem of hepatitis from a blood transfusion. Many people recall hearing about an American ambassador to Japan who, after an assassination attempt, received a transfusion in a Tokyo hospital and later developed hepatitis. Other public figures such as movie stars have been reported to have contracted the disease. The media have popularized the image of commercial blood banks collecting from storefront centers located in skid-row neighborhoods and frequented by drug addicts and alcoholics. It is in part from these images that a largely erroneous view has emerged and has been perpetuated in the public media that the hepatitis problem is determined by the payment that is received for a unit of blood, as if the disease were carried on the dollar bills used to pay the donors.

Laboratory testing for posttransfusion hepatitis is still far short of the capability to avert the disease entirely. Even the hepatitis B vaccine now undergoing clinical testing is unlikely to be routinely used to prevent hepatitis via widespread immunization of donors and prospective transfusion patients. Until the science and the technology evolve to the point of offering that capability, other approaches to the hepatitis problem are desirable. Discouraging payment for blood might well turn out to be a highly effective way to reduce hepatitis by screening out undesirable donors. However, the same effectiveness in reducing disease might be achieved if, instead of the blanket rejection of the concept of paid blood donation, blood banks were careful to select donors from pools of individuals meeting subjective and objective criteria of suitability. For example, one blood-bank director has recently decided to reject all donors who are unable or unwilling to provide a telephone number. Some blood banks have clearly become competent at a method of donor screening that permits both payment of some donors and low hepatitis rates.

Other Factors in Donation

Infectious Diseases

A number of other diseases caused by infectious agents are known to complicate the period following a blood transfusion. Some of these do not present major problems in the United States, because of effective screening techniques or low overall incidence.

Malaria has a low incidence in the United States, and, as a complication of a transfusion, poses little problem. However, in developing and tropical countries, there is a significant probability that a patient will receive blood contaminated with malaria. A history of malaria disqualifies a prospective blood donor for 3 years in the United States.

Syphilis is increasing in prevalence in the United States. Its causative agent can be passively transferred from an infective individual to a well individual. However, it is unclear whether the development of efficacious serologic tests for syphilis have had much effect in preventing posttransfusion syphilis. Some believe that the disease may no longer be contagious by the time that the serologic test for syphilis becomes positive.

Loss of Potency of Red Blood Cells

The two most commonly used blood preservatives, acid-citrate-dextrose and citrate-phosphate-dextrose with adenine, allow blood to be used for 21–35 days before it is considered outdated. The rationale for an expiration date for blood and its derivatives is twofold. First, it makes it possible to predict the potency of a particular unit. With increasing age, the red cells lose oxygen-carrying capacity. The oxygen-transfer potency of red cells as a function of age has been well studied and is readily predictable during the period of legal use. After that time, the potency is less certain and hence the blood is unacceptable for clinical use. A second justification for the dating of blood is an undesirable chemical change that takes place as blood ages: the alteration of pH and electrolyte composition. Blood preserved as a liquid becomes more acidic and accumulates potassium ions over time. The use of blood in which these changes may have taken place may upset pH and electrolyte balance in the recipient.

Donor-Recipient Blood Incompatibility

Antigen-antibody incompatibility reactions, sometimes with life-threatening complications, can occur even with ABO- and Rh-compatible donor-recipient combinations, despite the best efforts of the blood-bank staff. Strong incompatibility reactions occasionally occur as a result of interaction of minor antigen-antibody systems or because of antigen-related white-cell or platelet incompatibility.

One potentially avoidable cause of this kind of transfusion reactions is the mislabeling of blood. Little evidence is available on the frequency of labeling errors as a cause of incompatibility reactions. However, a recent study reported that fatal complications of transfusion accidents were being recorded at a rate of one death per million transfusions. Most fatalities were the result of transfusions given to the wrong patient.[30] How much other morbidity and mortality may have resulted is very difficult to assess. The error rate may lessen with the adoption of the machine-readable common bar code system of labeling that has been agreed upon in principle by the major blood-collection organizations as a result of the work of the Committee on Commonality in Blood Bank Automation and the Food and Drug Administration.

Consent for Transfusion

Gaining the informed consent of the patient for a transfusion at the time of admission to the hospital is common when blood use is anticipated. At that time patients are to be informed of the risks of transfusion therapy and are asked to sign a consent form. Hospitalized persons are unlikely to be able to evaluate the risk of complications of the transfusion against the potential benefits. The small number of patients who decline a transfusion that has been ordered by the attending physician are likely to do so because of religious beliefs.

Condition of Donor

A number of other protective practices are carried out for the purpose of avoiding compromising the health of blood donors by excluding those who, for medical reasons, can ill afford to part with a unit of their own blood. A full physical examination with extensive laboratory evaluation might be desirable, but accomplishing this for every prospective donor would prove expensive and impractical. Instead, criteria such as age, weight, blood pressure and hemoglobin concentration, and a general subjective assessment of how healthy the donor looks are used as surrogates for determination of who will be permitted to give. Guidelines and regulations for donor selection in the United States are conservative. The unwritten rule is to defer the donor if in doubt.

An experienced phlebotomist can often surmise from the appearance of the prospective donor whether or not the individual is in good health. An unhealthy person may threaten his or her own well-being by giving blood. Deferring a donor on the basis of general appearance is a judgment call, made on a subjective basis. Even prospective donors who pass the subjective criteria for general appearance may have reasons for exclusion.

In the healthy donor, the rate of synthesis of new blood cells and proteins increases after the donation in response to physiological signals that the blood volume and oxyhemoglobin content have fallen. The donor who is free of disease can be expected to replenish the supply of plasma protein within a few days. However, production of new blood cells to make up the deficit takes considerably longer. An individual's circulating blood is expected to be normal by the end of the eight-week period that American blood banks require before accepting the next one-unit donation. A donor is permitted to give blood at most six times per year in the United States. More frequent donation may be permitted in a few countries, but most allow fewer donations per year.

The resynthesis and resupply mechanisms for blood cells and proteins may be impaired in persons suffering from chronic diseases such as anemia. Blood hemoglobin level (one measure of anemia) and blood pressure (a measure of other chronic diseases) are examples of donor-evaluation criteria that are used to identify persons in whom a longer resupply time might be necessary. The minimum allowable hemoglobin level is 12.5 gram-percent for women and 13.5 for men. The range of acceptable blood pressures is 90–180 millimeters of mercury systolic and 50–100 millimeters of mercury diastolic.

Donation of a unit of blood causes the donor to part with cells, plasma, and proteins that make up about 10 percent of the circulating volume. The volume of a unit of blood is approximately 450 milliliters. Of this amount, nearly 55 percent is plasma and proteins. The quantity of circulating blood varies among individuals; body weight is considered to be a measure of total blood volume. In blood-bank practice, anyone weighing 110 pounds or more is assumed to have at least 10 pints of blood in circulation. Donors weighing less than this minimum figure may be permitted to donate proportionately less than a full unit. A smaller volume per donation is used in some other countries.

The rationale for age requirements (typically, that a donor be between 17 and 65; older with medical permission) is not nearly so specific as that for a minimum weight. It is based on the assumption that persons within this age range are more likely to be free of disease than those who are not. Recently the minimum age for donation in most places was changed from 18 to 17. High schools and other places frequented by teenagers are becoming important sites for blood collection. Teenagers may develop the "habit" of giving blood and continue to donate regularly as adults.

Blood Utilization: The Neglected Area of Quality Control

Nearly all of the efforts to control the quality of blood discussed so far are directed at the collection and transfusion services, the "supply side" of blood banking. The "demand side" has historically been left largely unchecked.

Current practice permits the physician who prescribes a blood transfusion for a patient to choose from a range of alternative products that might possibly be used to achieve the same therapeutic goal. Even when the choice of a particular blood product is not in doubt, the number of units ordered may be open to question. One unresolved controversy has surrounded the use of the single-unit transfusion. Many practitioners believe that little justification can be found for prescribing a single unit of blood. Their argument is that a patient whose problems are correctable with a single unit is not very different from a donor after a one-unit donation.[31] Others counter that donors are healthy subjects, but patients most likely are not.

The demand side of blood transfusion has been relatively free from quality-assurance efforts because it is so difficult to effect control in a professional group such as physicians. For certain blood products, the penalties that overutilization poses are those of economic inefficiency rather than patient compromise. In cases in which a patient's welfare may be threatened, liability would be difficult to assign because there are few standards of appropriate blood use. Reference 32 was a long-overdue attempt to profile patterns of blood utilization by practitioners. It is, however, a leap from having data on norms of usage and setting a standard.

If gaining agreement among practitioners about standards for blood use proves difficult, implementing them will also. Experience with peer review of practices among physicians has at best been mixed. Some hospitals and health-maintenance organizations report that "utilization review committees" have had success in reducing the lengths of hospital stays, but the federally mandated Professional Standards Review Organizations, which have provided peer review of physician's practices, have been seen by many as a disappointment. We still believe that greater attention to issues of quality and safety by those who order blood therapy would be worthwhile and could improve the quality of the transfusion experience.

The High Quality of Transfusion Practice

As transfusion practice has evolved over the past forty years, the natures of the risks to recipients and donors are much the same as they were in the beginning. The magnitude of those risks has, however, decreased significantly. Posttransfusion hepatitis and incompatibility reactions are still the major problems of compromise to recipients, and progress continues to be made in these areas. Specific efforts to protect donors are the object of continuing effectiveness review. More attention needs to be given to the criteria for blood therapy by those practitioners who prescribe it. Overall, blood transfusion is a relatively safe procedure in relation to its degree of technical complexity. The quality of blood-transfusion practice in the United States is, in general, quite high.

5 Nonprofit Organizations

The American National Red Cross and the American Association of Blood Banks (AABB) are the two major organizations collecting whole blood in the United States. Sharply different in structure and philosophy, they have been in conflict since the end of World War II for the control of the American blood-banking system. Three attempts at reconciliation have failed. Until a reconciliation occurs or one of the organizations becomes preeminent, blood banking in the United States will remain structurally divided no matter how well integrated are its medical aspects.

Just before the United States entered World War II, the Red Cross, at government request, accepted responsibility for collecting blood from civilian donors to fulfill the blood and plasma needs of the armed forces.[1] The significant advances in blood processing and transfusion therapies achieved during the war attracted the attention of civilian physicians and stimulated several scattered community hospitals and groups to begin collections of their own for local use. This relatively amicable division of labor—the Red Cross collecting blood for the military and local groups collecting for civilian needs—was not destined to survive for very long.

Primarily a disaster-relief agency, the Red Cross needs another mission to sustain itself between emergencies. Blood banking for civilian needs was consciously selected by the Red Cross as that sustaining mission at the end of World War II. But as the Red Cross sought to establish a national blood-banking system, its intended role in blood collections was challenged by the AABB, an association formed by hospital blood banks and community blood centers that had been established during or immediately after the war. The struggle for jurisdiction has heightened the philosophical differences between the organizations. The Red Cross defends a community-responsibility position, while the AABB defends an individual-responsibility position. With the recent movement toward all-volunteer donorship and the increased role of government in the financing of health care (including blood benefits), the conflict between the Red Cross and the AABB has intensified.

At the local level, however, the burdens of actually operating a blood-banking system are so great that the differing organizational philosophies have only limited meaning. Internal organizational strains are more important. Within the Red Cross the strain is between chapter volunteers and staff members and blood-banking professionals. Within the AABB the strain is between large blood centers and smaller (often dependent) hospital blood banks.

The Red Cross Program

The American Red Cross was founded in 1881 by Clara Barton, who had to struggle hard to adapt a European-developed concept of international charity to an America then very hostile toward foreign involvements of any type. In 1905 the Red Cross received a congressional charter to act as the chosen instrument by which the United States would carry out obligations assumed under the Geneva Convention for the protection of war victims, a convention the United States signed many years after it was proposed. The charter further obligated the Red Cross to act as the medium of voluntary services between the American people and the American armed forces and to provide a system of national and international relief to mitigate suffering caused by disasters.[2] Clara Barton's successor as president of the Red Cross, Mabel Boardman, established the Red Cross as a truly national organization in the early 1900s by creating a network of local chapters led by volunteers.[3] This combination of official responsibilities and voluntary action is both the strength and weakness of the American National Red Cross.

The test of the Red Cross's capacity to serve comes during national emergencies, especially wars. It is then that the Red Cross's ability to mobilize volunteers for public purposes is demonstrated. It is then also that the Red Cross is most exposed to criticism, for its performance tends to be judged by the public on the basis of its quasiofficial status rather than its voluntary organizational structure. The Red Cross has sought to avoid this vulnerability by maintaining a core professional staff and by stimulating voluntary participation during periods between emergencies. The core staff became the mechanism for channeling voluntary actions when they were required. The continual volunteer participation became the mobilization base for volunteer effort during emergencies. Inevitably, the Red Cross was drawn into a search for a sustaining mission other than war or disaster relief in order to keep its structure intact in times of peace and tranquility. Thus, the Red Cross came to teach water safety, to care for the elderly, and to visit the sick while waiting for catastrophe.

Given the degree to which Americans participate in voluntary charitable activities, it was inevitable that the Red Cross would come into conflict with other voluntary organizations that saw its potentially sustaining missions as their prime purposes for existence. Prior to World War I the Red Cross had the sale of tuberculosis stamps as one of its activities, but eventually gave way to the TB Society (now the American Lung Association). After World War I it offered services to wounded veterans, only to clash with the newly founded American Legion and Veterans of Foreign Wars. Red Cross first aid and swimming classes competed with instruction provided by the YMCA and the YWCA and many other organizations. Even Red Cross civilian disaster relief and aid programs for servicemen had rivals in the efforts of the Salvation Army, the Volunteers of America, the USO, and Army and Navy Relief.

Government also became a competitor, and a mighty one at that. After the 1930s and the New Deal, private charities could never hope again to match the resources for serious good works available to a federal government possessing an aroused social consciousness and backed by the tax code and a legion of civil-service professionals. Stricken Americans, be they the victims of flood, fire, or failing industry, increasingly learned that it was better to turn to the welfare state for succor instead of to charitable organizations such as the Red Cross.[4]

The wartime Red Cross, headed by Basil O'Conner, a prominent New Dealer and an intimate of President Franklin Roosevelt, was acutely aware of the problems private charities would face in the postwar years. The Red Cross's planning for the transition to peace began as early as 1943. It was not surprising that the successful new Red Cross program, the government-sanctioned franchise to collect blood for the war effort, would come to figure prominently in this planning.

Blood collection, this time for civilian use, seemed the perfect sustaining mission for the organization. As Foster Dulles, the Red Cross historian, put it, "It was believed that such a project represented an opportunity for service which would not conflict with government welfare work, would be of great value in the event of war as well as meeting the immediate needs of civilians, and was conspicuously in line with Red Cross idealism and experience."[5] No organization knew more about blood collections than the Red Cross; by the time the war ended the Red Cross would draw over 13 million units of blood for U.S. forces and their allies. Progress in the therapeutic use of blood and blood products appeared to ensure a growing demand. And there could be no better way to keep the Red Cross's name in the mind of the public upon whose support it depended than to have it involved in the "day-to-day emergency"[6] of blood collection.

During 1944 various groups, including the Association of State and Territorial Health Officers, the American Hospital Association, and the American Medical Association, were approached by Red Cross staff to determine their willingness to accept Red Cross management of the postwar civilian blood program. Favorable responses were received. Certain large unions had indicated their desire for the Red Cross to continue its involvement in blood collections. Assurances were obtained from the U.S. Public Health Service that it had no intention to establish a government-managed program.[7] Confident that there were no major jurisdictional obstacles to the establishment of a civilian blood program, the Red Cross's central managing board approved in April 1945 a staff recommendation calling for such a program.[8]

In essence two programs were approved. On the one hand there would be a *national blood program* based on the regional blood-collection centers created during the war with the assistance of certain large metropolitan Red Cross chapters. On the other hand individual Red Cross chapters of whatever size wishing to participate in blood collections could sponsor community-based donor-recruitment and even blood-drawing efforts with the approval of the Red Cross central office under what was called the *permissive blood program*. The Red Cross was undertaking a national responsibility that required central direction, but it was also a constituency organization that could not afford to hobble the initiatives of its many local chapters. This duality in the management structure of Red Cross blood collection was to be the source of constant friction and numerous reorganizations.

Endorsements of Red Cross involvement in a civilian blood-collection effort continued to be assembled during 1946 and early 1947. Eighteen regional meetings with chapter officers during this period produced a 97 percent approval rating from the 714 chapters represented.[9] A 1947 Gallup poll reported that 73 percent of the public favored a national blood program under Red Cross management, with 67 percent of those surveyed indicating a willingness to donate blood.[10] Formal initiation of the civilian blood program occurred in June 1947, when the Red Cross Board of Governors, the supreme policy-making body for the American National Red Cross, ratified the program design proposed by the Red Cross central staff.[11]

The goals the Red Cross set for itself were to have 81 centers open and collecting 310,000 units of blood per month within 3–5 years of the program's inception. The first center was officially opened in Rochester, N.Y. on January 12, 1948. Two years later, before the full impact on the Korean War mobilization had been felt, the Red Cross had managed to establish only 37 centers and a monthly collection rate of 80,000 units. The stimulus of the Korean War brought the numbers up to 44 centers and 127,000 units per month by December 1951, still far short of the initial goal.[12]

Part of this failure was due to overestimates by the Red Cross's medical advisers of the likely civilian need for blood. Not as much blood was needed as the Red Cross staff had been led to believe. The advisers, implying careful calculation, had originally stated that domestic blood demand would quickly grow to five units per year per general medical and surgical bed in civilian hospitals. Later they admitted that there were no solid data upon which to base such a figure.[13] The Red Cross also discovered that many of its chapters were unable or unwilling to raise on a continuing basis the funds required to support the blood program, even in cities where a major collection center was to be located.[14] Without the financial assistance of the local chapters the program could not expand, as the Red Cross had decided as policy that it would not sell the blood it collected. Worse yet, the Red Cross discovered opposition in many communities to its management of blood collections. What had been perceived as a popular activity certain to enhance the organization's national image was turning out to be a controversial undertaking miring the Red Cross in continuing conflict.

The American Association of Blood Banks

The Red Cross staff had assumed at the end of World War II that, if the Red Cross did not organize the civilian blood supply in the

United States, some other national organization or agency (the American Legion and the Public Health Service were mentioned) would do so.[15] Apparently not considered at the time was the possibility that local groups would believe themselves to be the appropriate custodians of their own community's blood resources. That hospitals, civic organizations, and even private entrepreneurs in some communities were already recruiting donors and drawing blood for local use had no visible effect on the plans prepared by the Red Cross for its civilian blood-collection program. Wartime collections had been intentionally limited to 36 centers in cities convenient to the few plasma-processing facilities then in existence. Apparently the Red Cross assumed that consultations with national bodies such as the American Medical Association and the American Hospital Association would ensure the local cooperation it needed in order to expand collections to the entire country and to remove potential competition.[16]

There was an awareness that the Red Cross was not universally liked. Its good works have not always been understood or appreciated by the public. A persistent belief is that the Red Cross somehow extracts profits from the charitable donations it receives. For example, rumors circulated in both the world wars that the Red Cross sold donuts and coffee to servicemen to enrich itself despite the intention of the millions who contributed money to the Red Cross during those wars. The Red Cross's explanation that the military sometimes forced the sale of such goods to American troops to avoid complaints from less-favored allied units or local entrepreneurs[17] never gained much public attention. Membership in the Red Cross varies from community to community, reflecting differential acceptance of the organization as a trusted and respected charity as well as differential willingness to be charitable. As was mentioned previously, the blood program was adopted by the Red Cross in part for its expected public-relations benefits. The hope was that, by doing obvious good, the Red Cross would gain general and continuing favor.

Almost immediately, however, the Red Cross began to encounter opposition to its self-proclaimed role as manager of all blood collections in the United States. Very few of the organizations that had established local blood-collection arrangements for civilian use during the war were willing to disband them or to otherwise assist Red Cross efforts in their areas after the war. Dozens of local medical societies openly challenged the legitimacy of Red Cross control, disregarding the endorsement the American Medical Association had given the Red Cross. In many areas physicians, hospitals, civic groups, and entrepreneurs moved to establish blood-collection arrangements, hoping to preempt the Red Cross. For some the possibility of making money in blood banking was the attraction; for others it was the opportunity to serve the community. Because these local efforts were unhindered by the Red Cross's need to coordinate national priorities with chapter predilections, they were often successful in staking out important jurisdictional claims. By the time the Red Cross program was formally inaugurated, large portions of the country, particularly in the Southwest and the upper Midwest, were already dominated by rival blood-collection agencies (ref. 16).

Representatives of many of these agencies, led by those from large blood banks in Phoenix and San Francisco, convened in Dallas in November 1947[18] to voice their opposition to Red Cross plans to organize the civilian blood-collection effort. An outcome of this meeting was the formation of the American Association of Blood Banks (AABB), the organization that was to champion the interests of local blood banks in national policy discussions.

Thwarting the Red Cross's ambition to become the total supplier of blood in the United States clearly has been one of the purposes of the AABB; becoming the scientific arbiter of blood banking has been another. Hematologists and pathologists have been active in the AABB because many independent blood banks are sponsored by or affiliated with hospitals, and hospitals usually allow their medical staffs to act as their representatives. As a result, accreditation of blood-banking facilities and the training of blood technicians have been important and highly regarded programs of the AABB. Because the Red Cross (much to the annoyance of its medical advisers) has tended to ignore or at least neglect the technical aspects of blood banking, the AABB has been able to use its scientific prowess to advantage in various public and governmental confrontations with the Red Cross.[19]

In keeping with its image as a scientific organization, the AABB opened its membership to individuals (for example, blood researchers and technicians) and to all blood-banking organizations, including the Red Cross and commercial banks. Though the Red Cross centers did not initially accept the invitation to join, several commercial banks did. Thus, the AABB has included in its ranks a small number of banks that pay donors and make a profit in supplying blood to transfusing units and processing agencies.

However, the dominant group within the AABB has always been the nonprofit blood-collection organizations—community blood centers and hospitals. Although some of these organizations, like all the commercial banks, did pay donors, most did not. Instead they relied on nonreplacement fees (typically $25–$50 per unit) as their prime incentive for donors. Some blood banks have required the recipient, or a relative or friend, to donate two or more units for every one used in order to avoid the fee. Nonreplacement fees actually collected are used for donor-solicitation advertising, equipment, and the other expenses of the collection organization.

The reliance on nonreplacement fees by many AABB members led in 1953 to the establishment, under AABB sponsorship, of the clearinghouse system. The clearinghouses, regionally distributed and now five in number, maintain records of an individual's or a group's blood credits and debits, thus facilitating the replacement of blood in times of need by relatives and friends distantly located. Periodically, the clearinghouse balances accounts among member banks, shipping blood from one center to another to clear accumulated paper indebtedness for units donated and transfused under the system.[20] The Red Cross participated in the clearinghouse system from 1961 through 1976 even though it did not sanction the use of nonreplacement fees or wish its blood to be shipped to proprietary blood banks. The clearinghouse system made the AABB a national organization, which forced the Red Cross to deal with it as an equal.[21]

In 1962 half a dozen of the larger blood banks, while retaining membership in the AABB, formed their own organization, the Council of Community Blood Centers (CCBC), in part to underline their hostility to the Red Cross but also to demonstrate their importance within the AABB. Through the years, however, the CCBC's positions on blood issues have changed considerably. Today, somewhat expanded in membership and representing nearly 20 percent of collections, the CCBC is usually a close ally of the Red Cross, strongly supporting the Red Cross's and the government's efforts to centralize blood banking into regions dominated by a single collection agency and accepting the notion that blood availability should be a community rather than an individual responsibility.

In contrast, the AABB has retained its stance as the defender of local blood banks and their interests. Formed during the intense postwar debate over national health insurance, the AABB resisted Red Cross attempts to "socialize" blood resources.[22] Today, in the face of increased government involvement in the regulation and financing of health-care services, it still champions the doctrine of individual responsibility in blood collections, stoutly defending the option of its members to use blood credits and nonreplacement fees.[23]

The Failures to Achieve Coordination

Three times in 30 years the Red Cross and the AABB have been brought together to design a framework for a cooperative national blood-banking program, under the assumption that blood-banking activities would be improved by the use of more uniform donation policies and common planning. Although the last of these coordination efforts is still being played out, the Red Cross and the AABB have by now clearly demonstrated an inability to reconcile their ideological and jurisdictional differences.[24]

The first of these efforts to achieve interorganizational coordination occurred in July 1950, when representatives of the Red Cross, the AABB, the American Medical Association, and the American Hospital Association met in Boston under the auspices of leading medical practitioners to discuss cooperation in blood collection. The resulting joint statement, the "Boston Agreement," called for a free exchange of blood between Red Cross centers and AABB member banks during peacetime and for the collection of blood for the military by AABB members in areas that lacked a Red Cross center during national emergencies.

Continuing tensions between the Red Cross and the AABB, and the outbreak of a real national emergency (the Korean War) that brought effective though temporary government-mandated coordination, soon rendered the Boston Agreement moot. The agreement, however, did hold significance for the Red Cross's National Blood Program. By meeting with the AABB, the Red Cross was admitting failure in establishing itself as the sole manager of the nation's blood supply. The Red Cross's National Blood Program now had an official competitor.[25] The next restatement of the purpose for the National Blood Program, issued in 1952, tacitly recognized the AABB banks as blood suppliers. The Red Cross would plan "to meet the *total or supplementary* civilian blood requirements of hospitals, physicians, and surgeons within the jurisdiction of Red Cross chapters which establish and operate blood programs in accordance with existing needs and local conditions" [emphasis added].[26] No longer did the Red Cross expect to be the sole procurer of blood for American medicine.

The American Medical Association acted as the broker for the second attempt to reconcile the Red Cross and the AABB, convening in 1954 a meeting of the participants in the Boston Agreement plus the American Society of Clinical Pathologists, the medical specialty group most concerned with blood banking. The outcome of the meeting was the establishment of the National Blood Foundation, which, when incorporated the following year as the Joint Blood Council, was to coordinate blood-banking activities in the United States.[27] Because the Joint Blood Council tended to confine itself to technical issues, such as devising collection standards and surveying existing practices, it had more staying power than the Boston Agreement. But because action required the consent of two-thirds of the Council's members (in essence this meant agreement between the Red Cross and the AABB, because of voting alliances with the other members), little of significance was accomplished.[28] The Council faded quietly away shortly after the Red Cross joined the Blood Clearinghouse Program in 1961, an event that seemed to symbolize a growing harmony between the major blood-banking organizations.

The harmony, such as it was, did not last long. The Red Cross was disturbed by attempts of the AABB in the mid-1960s to gain coequal designation as a manager of emergency blood collections for the military.[29] It also wanted an increase in the settlement fees for blood transactions processed through the clearinghouse system.[30] The AABB apparently was unhappy with the Red Cross's unwillingness to share responsibility for the entire national blood-collection effort and its chronic inability to meet blood demands in certain regions in which it was supposedly the dominant supplier. During this period the AABB successfully lobbied for the exclusion of the first three units of transfused blood from reimbursement coverage under the newly enacted Medicare program of federally financed health care for the elderly, thus protecting its nonreplacement-fee requirements and further exacerbating its relations with the Red Cross.

By the early 1970s the Red Cross and the AABB were again open antagonists. It was then that the American blood-banking system began to be subject to governmental review, largely as the result of Titmuss's *The Gift Relationship*. The variable quality, high waste rates, and other performance flaws of blood banking soon were documented in official reports[31] and became subjects of public discussion.

The federal government's response to the situation was to formulate in 1974 a national blood policy that called for vaguely specified improvements in the supply, quality, accessibility, and efficiency of blood resources and that was to be implemented, if possible, through voluntary, cooperative action (otherwise, the government threatened, it would exercise its regulatory powers).[32] The government's discussions with the major blood-collection organizations, including of course the Red Cross and the AABB, and interested medical groups to choose a private-sector instrument for implementing the government's blood-collection goals resulted in the proposal for the establishment of the American Blood Commission, the third attempt to create a mechanism coordinating blood collections in the United States.

In keeping with other federal policies, the Blood Commission has involved consumers as well as providers in the direction of its programs. Thus, representatives of the AFL-CIO, the American Heart Association, the National Hemophilia Foundation, the United Way of America, and other organizations now sit with the representatives of the Red Cross, the AABB, the CCBC, the American Medical Association, and the American Hospital Association on the Blood Commission. However, sharp divisions remain in the organization and management of the American blood-banking system.

Strains Within the Organizations

Although the jurisdictional conflict between the Red Cross and the AABB pervades national discussions of blood-banking policy, it has little relevance to local blood collection. There is little actual competition in blood banking. Except in a few metropolitan areas (Chicago and Houston are the prime examples), either the Red Cross program or an AABB or CCBC affiliate is the predominant blood supplier. At the local level it is intraorganizational strain rather than interorganizational conflict that is important.

The Red Cross and the AABB are constituent organizations; that is, they are composed of other organizations. Of the two, the AABB has the looser structure. Its members are nominally independent of one another, have separate local identities, and affiliate with the national association only as long as such an affiliation is convenient. The Red Cross's components are local chapters that depend on the national organization for their identification and, to a lesser extent, for their mission; their power within the organization comes from the fact that the Red Cross as now constituted cannot exist without their affiliation.

The internal strain within the AABB stems from the variation in scale among its 1,600-plus institutional members. Many of these members are hospitals that draw (if any) only a few hundred units of blood a year and have joined the AABB because the physician in charge of the blood bank (usually a pathologist) enjoys the professional identification that comes with membership or wishes to reward the bank's technicians with the opportunity to attend a convention in an exotic location. Other institutional members, far fewer in number, are regional blood centers drawing tens of thousands of units a year to supply dozens of hospitals and for whom blood banking is essentially the sole purpose. But no matter what the scale or regional role, each member institution has a single vote in determining AABB policy. It was this divergence in scale that, in part, caused several of the larger AABB members to form the Council of Community Blood Centers. Many of the smaller collectors were clients of these large institutions, and they used their AABB voting rights to express their resentments with being in a dependent position. Some of the larger AABB members, in turn, feel they have more in common with the Red Cross Blood Centers—only 57 in number and many quite large in terms of collections—than with hospitals belonging to the AABB that are really transfusers rather than collectors and processors.

The Red Cross's internal strains have their origin in the fact that the Red Cross blood program is an essential medical service superimposed upon a voluntary organization. Supplying blood to hospitals is a year-round, 24-hour-a-day responsibility involving coordination of donor recruitment, blood drawing, inspection, processing, inventory control, and delivery tasks. In contrast, the appeal of membership in a local Red Cross chapter for many volunteers lies in the social relations such membership offers: meeting once in a while with friends and neighbors, conferring status on one another through chapter elections, and doing some good at one's convenience or as the occasion requires. While volunteers may prefer organizing an annual first-aid training course or assisting in the relocation of fire victims, the blood program is committed to providing blood to meet the continuing needs of hospitals.

The structure of the Red Cross requires the blood program to depend heavily upon chapter support, which may or may not be forthcoming. Formation of a regional Red Cross Blood Center requires that a sponsoring chapter hold overall management responsibility for the operations of the center, but not one of the regional centers has its territory coterminous with that of its sponsoring chapter.[33] Nonsponsoring chapters may assist the centers in arranging local blood collections—but only on their own volition, because blood-donor recruitment (unlike disaster relief and service to the military) is not a mandated Red Cross activity. An additional 1,800 of the 3,100 Red Cross chapters participate in the blood program in this manner.

The dependence of the Red Cross blood program upon chapter support has important consequences. First, it permits much regional variability—some say too much—in what is supposedly a national program. The quality of leadership in the sponsoring chapter varies, as does the chapter's adherence to national Red Cross doctrines such as those governing the pricing of blood services and individual eligibility for blood. Second, it generates management tensions. There is often conflict between the regional blood centers and the sponsoring chapters and between the regional sponsoring chapters and the participating chapters. The National Red Cross exacerbates these tensions by forcing a dual lay and medical management structure on the blood program at each level. Thus, physicians, chapter managers, blood-banking professionals, and volunteers share in the operational direction of Red Cross–sponsored blood collections—not always harmoniously.[34] An additional problem is the fact that blood-banking personnel usually command higher salaries than do other Red Cross professionals, in recognition of their medical training and affiliations.

The financing of the blood program does not make relationships within the Red Cross any easier. Chapters sponsoring regional blood centers are expected to contribute to the maintenance of the program, which despite the processing fees for blood supplied to hospitals is not always self-sustaining. Nearly 60 percent of sponsoring chapters' expenditures are absorbed by the blood program. Nationally, blood program costs amounted to nearly $190 million in 1978—more than half of the total Red Cross budget in that year. Like other health-care costs, those for blood collection are rising rapidly.

Because it involves both fees and charitable donations, the financing of the Red Cross blood program is extremely complicated. The program has the potential to be entirely supported by the fees it charges hospitals, but such an achievement could threaten the financing of other Red Cross activities. The Red Cross is a participant in local United Way fund drives, which sometimes base their allocations to the Red Cross in part on the scale of that organization's blood collections. How willing the public would be to continue to support financially a Red Cross known to be covering all the expenses of its blood program, the most publicly visible Red Cross activity, through fees is a question some chapter staffs do not wish to contemplate. The failure to provide the blood program with all its financial requirements, however, can jeopardize the program's ability to meet the blood needs of the regions for which it has claimed responsibility. Uncertainty remains within the Red Cross about the desirability of expanding the blood program, despite its obvious importance.[35]

Many in the blood program recognize the limitations the association with the Red Cross places on their efforts. To them, blood banking is a bureaucratically structured, financially demanding activity that fits poorly within a voluntary organization. Attempts to assert control over sponsoring chapters through the use of the single national license the program possesses for all its regional centers have been ineffective in gaining desired reforms, as have the many management studies conducted for the program. It is not surprising, then, that the staff of the blood-banking program would consider more drastic steps to achieve organizational independence. In 1978 they proposed a joint venture with Baxter Travenol Incorporated for the large-scale commercial production of plasma fractions—a potentially lucrative but distinctly unprecedented undertaking.[36] Although the Baxter Travenol relationship did not materialize (because of many factors, including changing conditions in the plasma market and opposition within the Red Cross), its initiation gives evidence of the desire of many in the blood program to be permanently free from the vagaries of voluntarism.

6 Profit-Making Organizations: The Plasma Sector

A commercial blood sector exists side by side with the nonprofit sector. For the most part, the two are not in direct competition with one another. Nonprofit organizations specialize in the collection of whole blood and blood components, while commercial firms are principally active in plasma collection for the manufacture of blood derivatives. Unlike the voluntary sector, commercial blood banking has not been subject to government pressure for increased coordination. We now turn to this supposedly darker side of blood banking. Instead of a scandal-ridden underground, we find a sector that is filling an urgent need: supplying plasma and its derivatives to a world market. If our criteria for evaluating the performance of the commercial sector are adequacy of supply and quality of product, it seems that these criteria are largely being satisfied.

The Development of the Plasma Sector

The plasma sector is composed of the establishments that collect the plasma and the manufacturing firms that process it and bring it to market as blood derivatives or fractionated products. These two segments of the industry evolved largely independently; only recently has there been a trend toward the operation of plasma-collection centers by the blood-derivative fractionators.

When World War II created a greatly increased medical need for a safe and effective "fluid replacement" that could be used on the battlefield, researchers responded with the blood-fractionation technology, which made possible the production of derivatives that were stable in a variety of climates and easy to transport. Over time, civilian uses also became important.[1] A billion-dollar worldwide industry has grown to supply these new therapeutic products.

The development of the blood-fractionation technology was actually begun before the war. Edwin J. Cohn, head of the Department of Physical Chemistry at Harvard Medical School, began studies on protein fractionation in 1934 and was producing plasma derivatives from animals. There seemed little urgency to his work until threatening situations developed in Europe in the late 1930s and the U.S. Army began to anticipate large blood needs. The Committee on Transfusion of the National Research Council and the Medical Advisory Council of the American Red Cross asked Cohn to determine if animal plasma could be made safe for a human therapy. Within a short time, an animal-derived partial blood substitute was available for clinical tests. The side effects when animal derivatives were transfused into humans were not easily surmounted. Cohn and his group changed direction and began fractionating human blood. Arrangements were made for the American Red Cross to divert sufficient blood from its Boston affiliate to Cohn's laboratory for his research. The resulting "Cohn fractionation" technology yielded human plasma protein concentrate of high purity.

Clinical studies conducted through 1941 demonstrated the ability of certain Cohn fractionation products to restore blood volume in human volunteers without the same side effects that had accompanied the use of animal derivatives. However, clinical studies were still incomplete when the attack on Pearl Harbor took place in December 1941 and the United States entered the war. Human blood derivatives from Harvard were flown to Pearl Harbor and used in the treatment of injured servicemen. The National Research Council committee reviewed the consequences of this first military use as well as experimental data gained from clinical experience in domestic hospitals. Early in 1942 it recommended the regular use of plasma products by the armed forces. Later in 1942, construction began of commercial plant facilities for the large-scale production of Cohn fractions, with seven U.S. pharmaceutical firms cooperating under licenses granted under Harvard's patent.

Subsequent years brought only minor modifications in the Cohn fractionation technology. Not only has the Cohn process survived largely intact, but some experts have been critical of the fact that after nearly 40 years of use the products of blood fractionation are largely the same as they were in the early days of fractionation.[2] The Division of Blood Diseases and Resources of the National Heart, Lung, and Blood Institute in 1980 considered one of its priorities to be the development of new uses for and new products from the fractionation of human blood. The Institute has funded a number of investigators to conduct research in this area.[3] Throughout most of this period, the manufacture of blood derivatives and products has been capably monitored by the Division of Biologic Standards of the National Institutes of Health and its successor agency, the Bureau of Biologics of the FDA.

Also important to the evolution of the plasma collection and fractionation industry have been the commercial blood-collection establishments. Private firms have been a factor in U.S. blood collection for more than 30 years, nearly as long as blood banking has been practiced. For much of that time, the commercial blood collectors have been defensive about the role that they have played.

As early as the 1940s, commercial blood banks allowed themselves to be thought of as fulfilling the shortfall between needs and collection of the "more desirable" volunteer blood. A federal policy called "short supply" may even have legitimized this viewpoint. Under the short supply provisions, unlicensed commercial banks were permitted to supply blood to licensed collectors and processors when a needed item was unavailable.[4] In the 1960s, commercial blood banks increased the scope of their activities despite the increasingly prevalent view that the buying and selling of blood was to be discouraged. Though publicly in disfavor, commercial blood banks did well throughout the 1960s (particularly in the large cities), selling their blood to some of the most prestigious private hospitals and to many Veterans Administration hospitals.

Add to the problems of the commercial blood banks that they may have been dealing in contaminated product. Federal authority to require quality standards for blood collection was, throughout the 1960s, limited to those establishments engaging in commerce across state lines. Many commercial blood establishments restricted their activity to intrastate operations and thus escaped scrutiny by the regulatory agencies (only a minority of states maintained their own licensing or accreditation programs for blood banks).[5] When it was recognized that adequate safeguards may not have been taken to screen donors in many commercial banks, the contamination of commercially collected whole blood and components with hepatitis was first suspected and later documented.

Events of the late 1960s and the early 1970s gave greater public visibility to the actual and alleged shortcomings of commercial blood banking. The greatest public attention given this issue followed the publication in 1971 of Titmuss's *The Gift Relationship*, which was directly or indirectly responsible for the generation of numerous articles in academic journals and in the news media.

This media attention had its impact on the way blood is collected in the United States.

By the time the Department of Health, Education, and Welfare began work on its National Blood Policy in 1973 the number of commercial establishments collecting whole blood was insignificant. When it finally took effect in 1974, the National Blood Policy still did not provide for penalties to be applied against hospitals and other transfusion facilities that used commercial blood instead of unpaid blood.[6] A requirement to label blood as paid or volunteer was imposed by the federal government in 1978,[7] six years after a similar requirement was imposed by the state of Illinois and two years after labeling laws were enacted in California and Georgia. Hospitals were finding it more and more difficult to defend the purchase of blood from commercial banks, and by the end of the 1970s commercial whole-blood collection had all but disappeared.

To flourish or even to survive in blood banking, profit-making organizations needed a less publicly visible role. One such opportunity centered on serving the growing plasma-fractionation industry as wholesalers. By 1979, blood fractionators in the United States were being supplied with nearly 4 million liters of plasma, mostly by commercial collection establishments, for the manufacture of the increasingly popular therapeutic products of Cohn fractionation.[8] The plasma-collection facilities operating today, which are partly an outgrowth of the earlier commercial whole-blood-collection industry, include independent drawing centers as well as those owned and operated by the large fractionators.

Plasma Derivatives and Their Uses

Some information about the manufactured derivatives of plasma will provide a background for discussion of important issues facing the commercial sector and of the business of plasma. Table 6.1 identifies currently licensed human plasma products.

Blood derivatives manufactured from plasma can have therapeutic or diagnostic uses. The best source material is important to the generation of end products with a maximum of therapeutic value and a minimum of side effects. Lesser-quality raw material may suffice for the production of derivatives used as laboratory reagents for the diagnosis of certain diseases and conditions, when one need not be concerned about inducing disease

Table 6.1 Human plasma products licensed by U.S. Food and Drug Administration

---

Normal serum albumin

Plasma protein fraction

Immune serum globulin
Anti Rh globulin
Hepatitis B immune globulin
Measles immune globulin
Mumps immune globulin
Pertussis immune globulin
Rabies immune globulin
Tetanus immune globulin
Varicella zoster immune globulin
Vaccinia immune globulin

Antihemophilic factor
Fibrinolysin
Factor IX complex

Source: FDA regs. 21 CFR 600-799, April 1, 1980.

in a transfusion recipient. Therapeutic products are of greater interest economically to the commercial sector.

The principal therapeutic blood derivatives are the products of the Cohn fractionation process. First, plasma is separated from whole blood by sedimentation or centrifugation. Then, by a cold alcohol separation technique, it is broken down into groups of protein constituents called fractions. The fractions contain the important physiologically active protein products: albumin, immune proteins, and clotting proteins. For large-scale processing, plasma is first separated into a few major fractions and each one is then subfractionated under the conditions most effective for the further separation and isolation of the desired products.

Albumin

Early work on plasma fractionation centered on maximizing the yield of albumin, a highly effective expander of blood volume. Albumin has a large number of other clinical uses. As it can be used when not necessary without compromising the patient, such overuse often occurs (ref. 2; Randolph, ref. 1). Concern about overuse prompted a study, begun in 1975, whose objective was the development of guidelines for albumin's appropriate clinical use. The study named specific disorders for which regular use of albumin is justified: shock, burns, coronary bypass surgery, liver failure, and acute kidney diseases. A broad diversity of other pathologic complications were identified for which the occasional use of albumin was correct. However, the report of the study observed that for many other clinical disorders in which albumin is commonly prescribed there is incomplete or conflicting data on its effectiveness.[9]

Immune Proteins

The immune proteins or globulins confer protection in the form of circulating antibodies active against certain specific diseases. Referred to as the "gamma globulins," these preparations first became available toward the end of World War II. After the war several immune globulins were successfully developed and introduced for diseases such as measles, rubella, mumps, pertussis, tetanus, and vaccinia. Other immune globulins have become available more recently for prevention against hepatitis, rabies, varicella zoster, and maternal-fetal Rh incompatibility. The optimal preparation of immune protein derivatives makes use of blood from donors who either carry naturally or can be induced to carry high concentrations of specific globulins active against particular diseases.

Clotting Proteins

The freezing and controlled thawing of plasma results in the separation of cryoprecipitate, a substance containing the blood clotting factor missing in most patients who suffer from hemophilia. An important drawback of the clinical use of cryoprecipitate is that it requires very low temperatures, ice or dry-ice conditions, for preservation. In 1966, the first antihemophilic factor (AHF) concentrates were manufactured from plasma and commercially introduced. These new products were stable at higher temperatures, could be stored in refrigerators, and were more easily distributed. Additional protein clotting factors, a major advancement for the treatment of congenital bleeding disorders, became available as concentrates in the 1970s. AHF has seen the fastest growth in demand of all the plasma products.

The clinical use of plasma products is associated with less post-transfusion hepatitis than that of whole blood and blood components.[10] Albumin does not transmit hepatitis. Heat treatment of albumin at 60°C for 10 hours and consequent inactivation of virus is the presumed explanation. Immune globulins also are not responsible for the development of hepatitis; in fact they can protect against it. There has never been a good explanation for why immune globulins do not transmit the disease. (Reports of clinical hepatitis in recipients of immune globulins have been limited to cases in which nonstandard methods were used to prepare them.) AHF and other protein clotting derivatives can cause hepatitis. However, the usual recipients of these products, patients with hemophilia and other bleeding disorders, receive these agents routinely in transfusion. Surviving patients probably develop a high level of natural immune protection against hepatitis in response to continued exposure to antigenic stimuli in the AHF they receive. Hence, these products seem to be responsible for generating fewer clinical cases of disease than otherwise might be expected.

Revenue from sales of laboratory reagents derived from plasma and used to conduct *in vitro* diagnostic studies are becoming increasingly important to the plasma sector. Unlike the clinical products described above, these reagents are not administered in transfusion. The capability of diagnostic products to transmit hepatitis is of little consequence to patients, though it may increase the risks to laboratory workers.

The Collection of Plasma

With the growth in clinical uses for blood derivatives, the worldwide market for these products has been expanding. The demand for plasma, the raw material for the manufacture of blood derivatives, has become very large. Plasma collection in the United States is now approximately a $250-million-per-year industry.[11]

Most plasma is collected by for-profit firms that pay money to donors for the drawing of one or two units at a time. Public controversy has focused on the supposed exploitation of paid plasma donors in developing countries and in the ghettos of large American cities.[12] In reality, a broader spectrum of American donors have apparently become the dominant plasma suppliers to the world.

There are several alternative sources for plasma, some of which do not even involve active donation. Raw material for the manufacture of blood derivatives is classified as either "source plasma" or "recovered plasma," depending on its origin. Source plasma, the higher-quality material, is used to produce the major therapeutic plasma products and some diagnostic products. It is collected by plasmapheresis donation, or by whole-blood donation if the plasma is immediately separated from the red cells and frozen without preservatives. Until recently, source plasma also included that which could be extracted from placentas. Recovered plasma generally refers to plasma separated from outdated whole blood and red cells. The legal uses of recovered plasma are more limited than those of source plasma. Recovered plasma is permitted to flow into the plasma pool for fractionation of therapeutic products only under the short-supply provisions of federal regulations. It is principally used in the production of diagnostic reagents.

About 5.7 million liters of source plasma were collected during 1980 in the United States.[13] Nearly all of this plasma was obtained by commercial drawing centers using the plasmapheresis technique. According to an industry survey, 384 centers were supplying plasma to U.S. fractionators (see table 6.2). Of these, 381 were operating within the United States, one in Europe, one in Canada, and only one in a developing country (Belize, in Central America). As required by U.S. law, the domestic and foreign locations were all licensed by the U.S. Food and Drug Administration. Of the U.S. plasma-donation centers, 107 were operated by fractionation firms, 213 were owned and operated by multilocation firms that may have had other health-care products and services to offer but were not otherwise involved in blood banking, and 50 were independently operated single-location plasma-collection establishments. Red Cross regional centers and other community-based nonprofit collectors operated the remaining 11 establishments.[14]

Contrary to popular conception, the for-profit plasma collectors in the United States do not limit their operations to skid-row neighborhoods of large cities or change location every time their activities are "uncovered." Plasma centers exist in 30 states, with the largest concentration operating in California, Texas, and

Table 6.2 Plasma collection centers with U.S. licenses in 1979.

In United States	
Plasma-fractionator-operated	107
Independently operated multilocation companies	213
Independently operated single-location companies	50
ARC/community blood centers	11
	381
In foreign locations	4
Total	385

Source: "1981 Listing of Source Plasma Locations," *Plasma Quarterly* 3, no. 2: 53 (1981).

Florida, according to another 1979 industry survey.[15] Most of the centers are located in cities with populations of 500,000 or less. About 20 percent of the total were in the suburbs. Centers tend to be in business and professional areas and shopping centers. Over 70 percent of them have been in the same location for at least three years.

Of the three foreign plasma-collection centers holding U.S. licenses, the one in Europe is not currently supplying large quantities of plasma to U.S. manufacturers. The center in Belize provides American fractionators with an estimated 250,000 liters per year.[16]

As recently as 1976, U.S. fractionators were obtaining a much greater proportion of their plasma from foreign suppliers. One particularly large collection establishment, located in Nicaragua, was destroyed by fire in 1976. American news reports of the loss of the Nicaraguan collections brought to light the issue of obtaining plasma for domestic needs from underprivileged and possibly undernourished Third World donors who can ill afford to lose body protein. The closing of the center in Nicaragua also created acute concern among fractionation firms about the integrity of the plasma-supply network (ref. 13). Partly in response to these concerns, the trend toward acquisition of American plasma-collection centers by fractionators increased. As table 6.3 shows, by 1980 they were collecting 45 percent of their own source plasma. If ever the U.S. blood fractionators were heavily using foreign plasma sources to fulfill domestic plasma needs, the reverse is now the case.

Although the need for plasma derivatives may be comparable in the United States and Europe, domestic supplies of plasma in many foreign countries have not been nearly large enough to meet domestic needs.[17] To help meet the need of other countries, a large amount of U.S.-collected source plasma and U.S.-manufactured derivatives are now being exported. The United States is now the major world supplier of plasma products.

American firms developed their dominant role in plasma partly because of technological capability, but also because U.S laws permit the paying of plasma donors whereas those of several countries forbid it. In 1978 the Japanese company Green Cross acquired Alpha Therapeutics, a U.S. processsor with its own collection network—if not to secure supplies needed in Japan, then to increase Green Cross's share of the world plasma market. French and German firms have recently acquired fractionation and collection businesses in the United States, possibly for similar reasons. The French firm Institut Merieux bought North American Biological's plasma division in 1975, and the German firm Bayer acquired Cutter Laboratories in 1977. French law in particular forbids profiting from the sale and processing of human blood. Until the 1975 acquisition, Institut Merieux's supply of source plasma was limited to whatever they could extract from placentas obtained from

Table 6.3 Plasma sources of U.S. fractionators (excluding exports).

	Own centers	Contract centers
1978	35%	65%
1979	37%	63%
1980	45%	55%

Source: ref. 13.
a. The range among individual fractionators in 1980 was 30%–90%.

French hospitals. Institut Merieux has since sold its U.S. plasma operations to Biotest, a German fractionator. French blood-derivative manufacturers are now said to purchase partially fractionated derivatives from U.S. fractionators and to complete the manufacturing process and the marketing in their own country.

It is not true that a disproportionate amount of paid plasma collection in the United States takes place among minority populations. A Marketing Research Bureau study (based on a 3-month 1978 audit of 25 selected plasmapheresis centers throughout the nation, in which the records of 5,744 plasma donors accounting for over 30,000 donations were reviewed[18]) found that Caucasians accounted for 82 percent of the donations. Rejection rates for prospective commercial plasma donors were about 6 percent, as compared with typical 11–12-percent rejection rates among unpaid donors of whole blood in a Red Cross regional center.[19] Most rejections were because laboratory tests fell outside of normal limits. Very few people were prohibited from donating because their appearance or behavior failed to meet standards of acceptability.

Many commercial plasma donors undergo plasmapheresis on a regular basis. Most are paid $5–$20 for a session, in which they give 600 milliliters of plasma. Some individuals who carry rare antibodies needed for the production of certain hyperimmune globulins are paid much larger amounts and have earned thousands of dollars annually from plasma donation.

The short- and long-term effects of regular plasma donation by plasmapheresis on the health of the donors is a subject of current interest. There appear to be no short-term problems in healthy donors with adequate hemoglobin mass and serum protein levels. With proper dietary replacements and careful monitoring of donors, plasmapheresis seems to be a safe procedure for the collection of large volumes of human plasma over an extended period of time. Life-threatening complications of plasmapheresis have been encountered very seldom. The long-term effects of regular plasmapheresis donation are difficult to predict. The procedure emerged in the 1950s, became commonplace in the 1970s, and will need to be evaluated for several more years before the possibility of long-term complications can be ruled out. However, a number of physiological indicators suggest that this procedure may well prove to be safe in the long run, if appropriate safeguards are taken.[20]

The Plasma Business

Plasma fractionation is an international business with an annual sales volume of about $1 billion.[21] Some multinational firms that supply blood derivatives to the world market depend on plasma donations in the United States for their source material, but apparently rely on sales outside the United States for their profits.

Large-scale plasma fractionation is currently conducted in ten laboratories in the United States. Of these, the seven operated by commercial firms account for almost 95 percent of the production capacity. The remaining 5 percent of capacity resides in two state laboratories and a regional nonprofit blood-collection center. Table 6.4 identifies these fractionators and gives their actual manufacturing capacities (totaling over 4 million liters of plasma in 1979) and their estimated capacities for 1981.

Only three American-owned firms currently operate plasma-fractionation laboratories: Armour Pharmaceutical Company (owned by Revlon, Inc., a cosmetics firm that also is involved in other health-care products and services), Hyland Laboratories (a

Table 6.4 U.S. plasma-fractionation capacity.

	Plasma-fractionation capacity (liters)	
	1979[a]	1981[b]
Alpha	800,000	1,400,000
Armour	600,000	900,000
Cutter	1,200,000	1,700,000
Hyland	1,000,000	1,200,000
Massachusetts State Laboratory	50,000	50,000
Merck	100,000	—
Merieux–Biotest	100,000	100,000
Michigan State Laboratory	50,000	50,000
New York Blood Center	100,000	300,000
Parke-Davis–Immuno AG[c]	100,000	—
Total	4,100,000	5,500,000

a. Actual.
b. Estimated by Drees, ref. 8.
c. Parke-Davis's U.S. fractionation facility has been taken over by the Austrian firm Immuno; however, the future of its operation is uncertain.

division of Baxter Travenol, Inc., whose other products include plastic blood bags and intravenous solutions), and Merck, Inc. (a large pharmaceutical manufacturer). Merck was expected to cease its fractionation activities in 1981. Two other American-owned firms, Parke-Davis (which sold its plasma operations to the Austrian firm Immuno AG) and Squibb, had already left the business by 1981. Changes in FDA regulations announced in 1980 would have required those and other fractionators to commit large amounts of capital to meet new standards for plants and equipment.[22] The remaining commercial fractionation laboratories operating in the United States are at least partly foreign-owned, as mentioned above. The New York Blood Center (a nonprofit blood bank) runs a large fractionation laboratory, and two states operate smaller facilities.

As table 6.5 shows, the total capacity of fractionation laboratories in Europe to manufacture plasma derivatives was nearly 3.8 million liters of plasma in 1979, nearly the same as that in the United States. The European laboratories are reported to be functioning well below capacity because of difficulties in fulfilling their plasma needs (Drees, ref. 8).

The increasing acceptance of blood-derivative therapy is expected to lead to solid long-term growth for the plasma industry (ref. 13). In 1979–80, however, the industry experienced a downturn in revenues from plasma products as AHF was in the process of overtaking albumin. AHF concentrate is rapidly becoming the

Table 6.5 European plasma-fractionation capacity, 1979.

	Plasma-fractionation capacity (liters)
H. Behring, West Germany	750,000
Biotest, West Germany	100,000
Immuno, Austria	850,000
KABI, Sweden	250,000
Merieux, France	600,000
Red Cross, West Germany	375,000
Others (Netherlands, Finland, U.K., Swiss)	855,000
	3,780,000

Source: Drees, ref. 8.

leading plasma product (LeConcy, ref. 8; Randolph, ref. 1). Since World War II, albumin has been the most highly demanded product of fractionation. Fractionators used the observed demand for albumin as the most important determinant of how much source plasma needed to be procured. The recent worldwide acceptance of AHF for the treatment of bleeding disorders has caused the growth in demand for it to outpace that of albumin. The price of albumin declined 30 percent during 1979–80, while that of AHF increased. Manufacturers can now be expected to gear their fractionation toward maximizing the yield of AHF.

The profitability of the plasma-fractionation industry currently depends on sales of AHF—particularly on export sales of that substance from the United States to Europe, because the price per unit for exported AHF is much higher than its domestic price. A unit of AHF currently sells for $0.12–$0.16 in the United States, but can sell for $0.20–$0.60 in Europe. Table 6.6 provides an account of the major costs and revenues associated with the fractionation of 1,000 liters of plasma, in 1981 dollars, according to an executive from one of the leading fractionators. The costs of procuring and processing the plasma are estimated to be $70,000, exclusive of marketing and transportation costs. Revenues derived from sales of plasma derivatives (including AHF, albumin, and immune globulins) would

Table 6.6 Costs and revenues for fractionation of 1,000 liters of plasma.

Costs		
Procurement	$47,000[a]	
Fractionation	23,000	
Revenues		
	If AHF sold in U.S. at $0.12 per unit[b]	If AHF sold in Europe at $0.30 per unit[c]
AHF	$24,000	$60,000
Albumin[d]	33,000	33,000
Immune globulins[e]	6,000	6,000
	$63,000	$99,000

a. Liter of plasma assumed to cost $45, with an additional $2 for administrative costs.
b. Representative domestic U.S. price.
c. Representative price for material exported to Europe.
d. Assumes that albumin is sold for $1,500 per kilogram.

total only $63,000 and would lead to a shortfall if the AHF were sold at lower unit prices such as those common in the United States. If the AHF were exported to Europe and unit prices remained high, revenues could be nearly $100,000 and thus could reflect a profit, even after distribution and marketing. However, the upward price pressure for AHF in the United States and the downward pressure in Europe may make it impossible to maintain a large differential in prices.

The Future

As we have seen, the profit-making organizations in blood banking's commercial sector have evolved to perform an important service in a manner that appears to be in the public interest according to the criteria of adequacy of supply and quality of product. The commercial sector has for the most part been compliant with the increasingly stringent "good manufacturing practices" for blood products that have been promulgated by the FDA. Their continued dominance in plasma would be threatened only by the possibility of competition from the voluntary sector or by government-mandated elimination of payment for plasma donors.

In the United States, the nonprofit sector shows little interest in managing the collection of plasma on a large enough scale to fill the needs of the blood-derivative manufacturers. Plasmapheresis collection depends on donors' willingness to spend up to 2 hours or more until the process is completed and has not been successful in generating adequate plasma supplies in many countries where a voluntary agency has the exclusive franchise.

Nonprofit blood centers could find plasma collection more attractive if new technology were available to reduce the time required to make a plasmapheresis donation to about the same as for a whole-blood donation. Automated plasmapheresis equipment, including some models that make use of new fast membrane technologies, is already being exhibited at professional meetings. However, according to one analyst, the new technology will not in the near future prove cost-effective for use in the United States, because the cost of disposables is high, because plasma donations will still take longer than whole-blood donations, and because the commercial plasma centers using manual methods can still do it all for less.[23]

Large-scale plasma fractionation appears to be even less attractive to the nonprofit sector. The American Red Cross and two state laboratories have been fractionating small amounts of plasma for a number of years. However, the Red Cross contracts with major U.S. commercial fractionators and with nonprofit laboratories throughout the United States and Europe to process most of the plasma collected by its regional centers into blood derivatives. Nonprofit plasma fractionation has been limited to only a few percent of the total capacity. A proposed joint venture in which Baxter-Travenol and the Red Cross would have jointly operated a fractionation facility that might have brought them as much as 30 percent of the world market for blood derivatives was canceled, apparently because both parties questioned whether the benefits that were likely to emerge from such an arrangement were worth the costs in dollars and in public and industry relations.

Given that the plasma collection and fractionation industries have become well established and the nonprofit sector does not seem to want to take over their functions, we believe it unlikely that the U.S. government will move to eliminate payment for plasma donors. When the National Blood Policy, which mandated the elimination of paid whole-blood donation, was announced, it was implicitly assumed by many that similar efforts would be directed toward the plasma supply in the future. However, the current system of plasma collection and processing appears to work reasonably well, and there seems little justification for tampering with it.

7   Attitudes and Decisions About Donation

Much of the talk about the blood supply emphasizes the alleged difficulty of setting an adequate number of people to give blood. Messages from the collection organizations suggest that, in spite of their relentless efforts, the blood supply hovers perilously close to panic levels. Literature on donor motivation and recruitment laments that so few people (about 3.5 percent of the population, or about 10 percent of those eligible to donate) give blood each year.

We noted above that the present needs for whole blood and red cells (but not blood pharmaceuticals) require, on the average, one whole-blood donation from every eligible potential donor about once every seven years. In this chapter we argue that the seemingly small number of people who give blood in any one year results from the limited need for whole blood rather than from unwillingness of the public. Our data provide a more respectful and appreciative perspective on the public's attitudes and decisions with regard to blood donation.

There is a large literature on blood-donor motivation and recruitment, overviews of which have been presented by Oswalt.[1] Most contributions to this field have been limited in scope. Representative topics include comparisons of people who do and who do not participate in the blood supply, the relevance of an individual psychological effect for the motivation and/or retention of blood donors, and public attitudes toward the two major blood-collection ideologies, community and individual responsibility.

Almost all such work is performed in cooperation with a single blood program. Little recognition is given to the degree to which the population studied may have been conditioned by the viewpoints of the local collection programs. Most of the literature on motivation and recruitment reflects, either implicitly or explicitly, three common sets of assumptions about the blood supply:

- that the blood supply is marginal at best, more blood is always needed than is collected, and the timing and selection of medical procedures are affected too often by blood shortages,
- that great reluctance to donate blood on the part of most people is the critical impediment to the improvement of the blood supply, and

- that, in deciding whether, when, and where to give their blood, potential donors are choosing among alternative "reasons" for giving and among the alternative collection organizations that provide these reasons, and therefore it is vital that we learn which ideologies, reasons, and collectors result in the most satisfactory blood collections.

In chapter 1 we indicated that the performance of the blood supply is vastly better than its reputation. As a result of work to be reported on in this chapter, we also do not agree with the second and third of these assumptions.

The information on whole-blood collections and on the nature of public participation in the blood supply[2] is less substantial than one might expect. (Gradual but important improvements are evolving from the National Blood Data Center established by the American Blood Commission in Arlington, Virginia.) This chapter draws upon research conducted by Alvin W. Drake under the sponsorship of the National Center for Health Services Research.[3] The work included comparative studies across several distinct blood-collection environments.

A Study of Attitudes and Decisions

The objective of our project was to obtain a more complete understanding of several practical aspects of public attitudes and decisions with regard to blood donation. Study topics included the degree and nature of participation in the blood supply, perceptions of and personal "closeness" to blood needs, nondonors' and donors' perceptions of the blood supply and of donation opportunities, how ex-donors come to achieve that status, and attitudes with regard to blood-collection ideology.

Our resources permitted us to design, pretest, and conduct surveys on a significant scale, often using identical survey instruments in several different collection environments. Some efforts were directed at special groups, such as ex-donors, very frequent donors, people whose workplaces provide an intense blood-collection environment, and high school students at the time of their first convenient donation opportunity.

Selection of the actual survey research design to be used involved both theoretical and pragmatic issues. Some of our interests required the cooperation of large centralized blood-collection programs that would have, in accessible form, the detailed donor records needed for us to pursue particular topics. Other interests required access to special populations such as those mentioned above. Our final and most expensive survey work (the "general-public" activity described below) required a set of metropolitan areas with significant but understandable differences in their blood-collection systems. The data presented in the following sections come primarily from our final, general-public survey. We also refer to some results from two other major surveys and from one less carefully controlled pretest activity.[4] Brief overviews of these four survey research activities follow.

General-Public Survey

Telephone interviews (about 20 minutes each) were performed with samples of the general public in the 17–65 age group. The interviews were preceded by mail contact with the selected households. If required, many callbacks were made to reach the statistically selected respondent for each household. Interviewers were available with competence in all common foreign languages. About 460 households responded, providing a response rate of about 80 percent. This work was performed in the Hartford, Houston, and New York metropolitan areas, which were selected for their diversity in blood-collection ideologies and practices.

Survey of Insurance Company Employees

Questionnaires were completed by several groups of employees at each of three large insurance companies in the Hartford area. The questions were very similar to those used in the general-public survey. About 510 employees participated, providing a response rate of about 98 percent. The companies were selected because they provide the most intense nonmilitary blood-collection environments of which we are aware. Employees are provided regularly with blood information, solicitation, and frequent, convenient blood donation opportunities. Unlike most of the U.S. population, people who work at these insurance companies are almost forced to form explicit, nonconjectural attitudes about blood donation. The blood information and collection programs at these companies have existed in their present form for many years.

High School Survey

Questionnaires were completed by students at four high schools in Massachusetts shortly after most of those students 17 years or older were confronted with their first convenient opportunity to give blood. About 2,000 questionnaires were completed, providing a response rate of about 90 percent.

Survey of Frequent and Former Donors

Questionnaires were completed at home by target populations of unusually frequent donors and by people who appeared to have stopped making blood donations. Potential respondents were mailed questionnaires after being selected from the records of the central blood programs in Bergen County, N.J., and in the Hartford, New York, and Minneapolis metropolitan areas. Letters encouraging participation were sent by officials of the local blood program. About 365 frequent donors and about 215 apparent ex-donors participated, providing response rates, respectively, of about 55 and 30 percent. This survey activity was one of our pretests, directed toward understanding the relationship between the ideologies of blood programs and the ideologies of their donors and toward seeking out some of the differences between active, frequent donors and people who appear to have stopped donating.

The general-public, insurance company, and high school surveys were performed in the late spring and early summer of 1976. The survey of frequent and former donors was performed in the fall of 1975. We are aware of no developments that suggest that the character of the survey responses would have been significantly different if the activities had been repeated five years later.

All surveys, including ours, suffer from significant methodological limitations. For the work at hand, we wish to note some additional limitations and a few advantages.

Even simple matters of fact, such as the general details of a person's entire blood-donation history, may be unknown to the donor and to the collection organizations. Name changes and incomplete recordkeeping within a collection program may make it difficult or impossible for the program to ascertain the number of donations it has received from an individual during even the most recent three or four years. Given also the general mobility of the population and the fact that donors may have received and discarded several donation cards from one or several blood collectors, we conclude that there will be considerable uncertainty associated with all estimates of individual donation histories.

Even greater limitations apply to all attempts to characterize attitudes toward blood-collection ideology and policy, topics likely to be low on any person's list of items for thought. Existing studies performed by the major collection organizations do not help much, because the desired results of a study may have been clear long before the data were collected. For example, one collection organization may claim to assess public opinion by asking whether "the family and associates of a patient should have the right to assist with blood replacement." Another organization, seeking a different result, may ask whether "the family of the patient should carry the additional burden of blood replacement." These are only mild caricatures of the items with which the AABB and the Red Cross have set out to document public preferences between individual and community responsibility. We did what we could to prepare more neutral survey items.

The scale of our activities offered many advantages over earlier studies on related topics. A number of pretests allowed us to sort out the issues and to develop survey items that were relatively clear and neutral. Within a single survey instrument, we were often able to approach an important issue from several points of view. For example, in order to determine whether an ex-donor achieved that status consciously, we included at various places in the survey instrument items such as these:

Was anything either especially good or bad about your most recent donation experience?

Have you heard anything favorable or unfavorable about blood-collection organizations since your last donation?

In the last few years, have there been any changes in your opportunities for blood donation?

In the last few years, have there been any changes in your blood-donation eligibility?

How many blood donations do you anticipate making in the next two years?

The responses to an entire set of items similar to these allowed us to conclude, with considerable confidence, that most ex-donors acquire that status because of externalities rather than by any conscious choice. Other sets of survey items allowed us to assess the consistency of an individual's attitudes toward individual and community responsibility.

The tables in this chapter are based on the responses to the surveys. Often we concentrate on comparative rather than absolute uses of the data obtained. Whenever appropriate, survey items are quoted or paraphrased in the tables that present their results. The complete survey instruments are included in our project reports.

Perceptions of Blood Needs

Do people underestimate the importance of the blood supply? Are blood needs primarily an abstract concept for most people, or have most people had personal experience with patients who have needed blood?

Blood bankers insist that the public is altogether too unaware of the need for blood. Much of the literature on donor recruitment conveys the assumption that perceptions of the need for blood provide an important distinction between donors and nondonors. Similarly, the initial deliberations of the American Blood Commission assumed that improving public education about blood needs could do much to alleviate present problems with the blood supply.

As one measure of personal involvement with blood needs, we asked people whether they, a relative, or any other personal acquaintance had ever received a blood transfusion. The salient feature of the data in table 7.1 is the surprisingly high degree to which people have had personal contact with blood needs and use. This is among the reasons why we have come to doubt that remoteness of the concept of blood needs constitutes a serious limitation on the blood supply.

Table 7.2 presents several measures of the perceptions of blood needs held by people with different degrees of participation in the blood supply. To focus on the issue of interest, we include in the first column data only for those nondonor respondents who consider themselves eligible to give blood. The people who have made more blood donations, of course, tend to be somewhat older. They are also more likely to know somebody who needed blood. However, for the variety of measures used here, perceptions of the need for blood are not a major factor in separating the

Table 7.1 "Personal closeness" to blood needs.

Age group	n	Percentage "close" to blood needs
17–20	26	39
21–30	101	51
31–40	98	76
41–50	76	83
51–60	72	81
61–65	48	80
All	421	70

Survey activity: general public.
Population represented: all respondents.
Note: A respondent is said to be "personally close" to blood needs if he, a relative, or another personal acquaintance has received a blood transfusion.

Table 7.2 Perceptions of blood needs.

	Number of donations		
	None, but eligible	1–3	≥4
n	141	88	106
Percentage of group that is "close" to blood needs	58	77	81
Average index for chance a person will need blood	3.04	3.09	3.13
Average index for chance a hospital patient will need blood	2.65	2.60	2.73
Average index for adequacy of local blood supply	1.96	2.02	2.01

Survey activity: general public.
Population represented: eligible nondonors and all donors.
Displayed: average indices for the scales below.
Indices: For number of people out of 1,000 who will need blood sometime in their lives, 1 in 1,000 = 1, 10 in 1,000 = 2, 100 in 1,000 = 3, 300 in 1,000 = 4. For percentage of people admitted to hospitals who will require blood transfusions, about 5% = 1, about 10% = 2, about 25% = 3, about 50% = 4, about 75% = 5. For impression of the adequacy of the local blood supply, "usually adequate" = 1, "occasional shortages" = 2, "frequent shortages" = 3, "continual crisis" = 4.

three classes of respondents (eligible nondonors, people who have made 1–3 blood donations, and people who have made more than 3 donations).

Although our samples could not be made large enough to control for all factors, such as the age and sex of people with different degrees of participation in the blood supply, our data do support two important conclusions: that personal experience with blood needs is broadly distributed among the population, and that perceptions of blood needs are not very different among people who do and those who do not give blood.

We also find that a highly informed population, such as the insurance company employees, describes the adequacy of the local blood supply in much the same way as does the general public in the same region. The more frequent solicitation and the convenient donation opportunities, rather than differences in perceptions of blood needs, account for the fact that these insurance company employees give much more blood than do their counterparts in the general public.

Solicitation and Opportunity to Donate

With the exception of responses to acts of nature and to highly publicized individual blood needs, few people are inclined to go far out of their way to give blood. We expect a person's degree of participation in the whole-blood supply to reflect the person's exposure to solicitation efforts and to convenient donation opportunities. In this section, we consider some elementary data on the outreach of the blood-collection system.

Participants in the surveys of the general public and of the insurance company employees were asked several questions about solicitation and about donation convenience. Although a request to replace blood for a particular patient is strong motivation for donation, we concentrate on more common forms of solicitation; individual blood-replacement requests are not considered in the data discussed here.[5]

Tables 7.3 and 7.4 present simple descriptions of the extent of solicitation and the donation opportunities for the general public and the insurance employees, respectively. Participants are grouped by degree of participation in the blood supply in the same manner as in table 7.2. We are not surprised by the great

Table 7.3 Solicitation and donation opportunity, general public.

	Number of donations		
	None, but eligible	1–3	≥4
n	141	88	106
Percentage of group asked, in person or by telephone, to donate blood (other than for a particular patient)	19	38	54
Percentage of group that now has a convenient time and place to give blood regularly	54	60	72

Survey activity: general public.
Population represented: eligible nondonors and all donors.

Table 7.4 Solicitation and donation opportunity, insurance companies.

	Number of donations		
	None, but eligible	1–3	≥4
n	117	127	136
Percentage of group asked, in person or by telephone, to donate blood (other than for a particular patient)	78	82	85
Percentage of group that now has a convenient time and place to give blood regularly	83	94	99

Survey activity: insurance companies.
Population represented: eligible nondonors and all donors.

intensity of solicitation and the convenient donation opportunities for the insurance employees; our anticipation of such results was the basis for our decision to use these companies to represent an intense blood-collection environment. For the general public, the correlation between solicitation and donation in table 7.3 is of the form one would anticipate. However, for three different metropolitan areas with a great variation in the organization of blood-collection arrangements, the fraction of the people who believe they now have a convenient time and place to give blood regularly is remarkably high. One could argue, in fact, that if a broader donor base were actually needed these convenient donation opportunities would have been extended to the people who do not yet receive them.

We also learned that, in all three metropolitan areas included in our work with the general public, eligible nondonors tend to be slightly more supportive than nonsupportive of the statement "More pressure should be used to get people to give blood." One is inclined to believe that additional solicitation and/or improved convenience of donation opportunities is all that would be required to convert some of these eligible nondonors into donors. As we will discuss below, the same is certainly not true for the eligible nondonors at the insurance companies. In the intense blood-collection environment, maintaining one's nondonor status requires a deliberate decision not to donate.

The outreach of present donation opportunities is quite broad. It would have been surprising if the factors considered in this section had not correlated with a group's participation in the blood supply.

Actual and Perceived Eligibility

Various types of medications, medical conditions, and exposure to certain diseases are among the factors that may make an individual temporarily or permanently ineligible to give blood. Our own work and other data available in the literature suggest that, by and large, members of the general public tend to overestimate their eligibility for blood donation.

Data based on health statistics and medical eligibility requirements lead to an estimate that, at any particular time in 1976, about 75–80 million people in the United States were eligible to give blood.[6] Table 7.5 presents data from an item about perceived

Table 7.5 Perceived eligibility.

Age group	Males		Females		All	
	n	Percentage perceived eligible	n	Percentage perceived eligible	n	Percentage perceived eligible
17–30	58	88	75	77	133	82
31–40	50	88	49	47	99	68
41–50	30	87	47	55	77	68
51–60	35	71	37	59	72	65
61–65	20	50	28	46	48	48
All	193	81	236	60	429	69

Survey activity: general public.
Population represented: all respondents.
Displayed: percentage of respondents in each group who believe they are "medically eligible to give blood now."

eligibility that was part of our general-public survey. About four out of every five male and about three out of every five female respondents judged themselves to be eligible for blood donation at the time of the survey. Applying their responses to the population and the age distribution of the United States in 1976, we obtain an estimate that about 85–90 million people in the United States considered themselves eligible to give blood at that time.

Even though the quality of these estimates is limited by the sample size and by some oversimplifications in the methodology, it does seem reasonable to conclude that for each of the about 10 million units of whole blood collected in 1976 there were about eight people who considered themselves medically qualified to donate it. It seems unlikely that either actual medical eligibility requirements or individual perceptions of these requirements constitute significant limitations on the adequacy of the whole-blood supply.

The Distribution of Donors in the Population

We have indicated our belief that it is the limited need for whole blood, rather than the willingness of potential donors to part with their blood, that explains why "so few" people (actually about 8 million in 1981) give blood. In this section, we present data on the degree to which participation in the whole blood supply is distributed in the population.

We begin by summarizing some results from our general-public survey of samples of people in the age group for regular blood donation (17–65 years) in the Hartford, Houston, and New York metropolitan areas. About 44 percent of these people reported that they had made at least one blood donation. Of the people who considered themselves eligible to donate at the time of the survey, 53 percent reported at least one donation. Although one can think of several sources of error in using these results to characterize the fraction of all people in the 17–65 age group who have given blood, it appears safe to conclude that the experience of blood donation is broadly distributed in metropolitan populations. Furthermore, data from the 1973 National Health Interview Survey indicate only slight differences in blood-donation activity between urban and rural populations.[7] Our results contrast severely with common statements about how few people have participated in the blood supply.

In table 7.6 we display the percent of males and females in each age group who indicated having participated in the blood supply at least once. About 60 percent of all male and about 30 percent of all female respondents report one or more donations. Females are somewhat more likely to be ineligible and significantly less likely to have convenient donation opportunities. Note the remarkably

Table 7.6 Participation in blood supply.

Age group	Males		Females		All	
	n	Percentage who have donated	n	Percentage who have donated	n	Percentage who have donated
17–30	58	43	75	24	133	32
31–40	50	66	49	20	99	43
41–50	30	80	47	38	77	55
51–60	35	69	37	43	72	56
61–65	20	55	28	25	48	38
All	193	61	236	30	429	44

Survey activity: general public.
Population represented: all respondents.

high participation rates reported by males within the 31–60 age group. These figures are especially impressive when one recalls that the respondents include some people who have always been ineligible, some people whose failure to donate may result from a temporary rejection at their first donation attempt, and a significant number of people who may have experienced little or no serious solicitation.

Some data on recent participation in the blood supply are given in table 7.7, which concerns participants who considered themselves eligible to give blood. In this table we display, within age groups, the percent of the respondent population that reported at least one blood donation during the previous 3½ years.[8] Once again we find evidence of broad public participation in the whole-blood supply, with 31 percent of the males and 22 percent of the females reporting at least one blood donation within the most recent 3½ years.

The distribution of the total number of blood donations reported by respondents in the general-public survey is given in table 7.8. About 20 percent of the donors (or 9 percent of all respondents) had made only a single donation, and about 22 percent of the donors (or 10 percent of all respondents) reported more than ten donations. For an adequately large sample of respondents,

Table 7.7 Recent participation by people who believe they are eligible.

Age group	Males		Females		All	
	n	Percentage who donated in last 3½ yrs.	n	Percentage who donated in last 3½ yrs.	n	Percentage who donated in last 3½ yrs.
17–30	51	33	58	21	109	27
31–40	44	27	23	22	67	25
41–50	26	27	26	27	52	27
51–65	35	34	35	20	70	27
All	156	31	142	22	298	27

Survey activity: general public.
Population represented: eligible respondents.
Displayed: percentage of eligible respondents who believed they had given blood at least once during the last 3½ years.

Table 7.8 Total donations per donor.

Total no. of donations	Percentage of respondents ($n = 424$)
0	57.3
1	9.0
2	5.9
3	4.2
4–5	7.1
6–10	6.6
11–20	6.1
> 20	3.8

Survey activity: general public.
Population represented: all respondents.

data like this become much more informative when people are grouped by age and sex. Although some of this is done in our project reports, only the eventual tabulation of the data from the 1978 National Health Interview Survey will provide definitive information.

As an additional example of the degree of public willingness to participate we include table 7.9, which concerns one aspect of our studies of high school blood collections. In this table we consider only students who were at least 17 years old and who did not think of themselves as permanently ineligible to give blood. About 26 percent of these students gave blood in response to what was, for most of them, the first realistic opportunity. Another 25% apparently made a reasonable effort, but were unable to donate either because their parents would not sign a consent form (required for people at age 17 in their state) or because they were designated at least temporarily ineligible at the donation site. Only about half of the students said that they did not try to donate.

Data given in the present section provide some strong examples of the basis for our belief that public willingness to participate in the blood supply is far greater than the blood-collection organizations will ever admit. We think it conservative to estimate that there are more than 40 million experienced blood donors in the United States, about 30 million of whom are medically eligible and most of whom are ready and willing to give again under reasonable circumstances of solicitation and opportunity.

Table 7.9 Participation in high school blood drives.

	Males (n = 98)	Females (n = 103)	All (n = 201)
Tried to donate and succeeded	31.3%	22.7%	26.5%
Tried to donate and failed[a]	14.8%	33.0%	25.1%
Did not try to donate	53.8%	44.2%	48.6%

Survey activity: high schools.
Population represented: students 17 years of age or older who did not consider themselves permanently ineligible and believed they had had at least one convenient donation opportunity.
a. This category consists of students who were declared ineligible at the donation site and students who were 17 years of age whose parents would not sign the required permission forms.

Attitudes and Reasons of Nondonors

We use the term *nondonor* for people who say they have never made a blood donation. This section considers nondonors' attitudes toward blood donation and their "reasons" for not participating in the whole-blood supply. We concentrate on nondonors who consider themselves medically eligible for blood donation. As one would expect, there are major differences between the attitudes of nondonors in the general public and nondonors in the intense blood-collection environment at the insurance companies.

In our work and in the rest of the literature, three responses dominate all others when eligible nondonors are asked why they have never given blood. The common types of responses are "Nobody asked me," "I never thought about it," and "There was no convenient opportunity." Early in our general-public questionnaire, before other items that might suggest possible reasons, we included an open-ended inquiry as to why eligible nondonors had not given blood. Because many replies were phrases essentially identical to those used in table 7.10, the verbatim responses were unusually easy to group. Many of these nondonors may have had little reason to think seriously about blood donation. A few had had bad experiences when they had tried without success to give blood. The three common reasons noted above plus various forms of fear account for about 67 percent of the responses. Some combination of being asked, thinking about donation, and having a convenient opportunity would convert some of these nondonors

Table 7.10 Distribution of open-ended reasons for nondonation.

	Percentage of all responses from		
	Males ($n = 55$)	Females ($n = 86$)	All ($n = 141$)
Never asked	18	18	18
No convenient opportunity	17	17	17
Fear	11	21	17
Never thought about it	20	11	15
No real need	11	7	8
Bad previous experience	5	2	3
Other	18	24	22

Survey activity: general public.
Population represented: eligible nondonors.
Displayed: percentage of all nondonation reasons coded into the given categories.
Notes: For cases in which a respondent provided two reasons, each was given a weight of ½ reason for purposes of this tabulation. Responses to the open-ended request for the respondent's reasons for nondonation are listed for various nondonor groupings in technical report 136 of the MIT Operations Research Center.

into donors. It would also, of course, remove much of the conjecture from these nondonors' attitudes toward giving blood and, over time, firm their positions one way or the other. Similar information, obtained from a survey item asking for ratings of potential reasons for nondonation, appears in tables 7.11 and 7.12. Of the reasons for not donating used here, not having been asked personally consistently achieved the highest ranking. At least after averaging over all eligible nondonors, no reason comes close to a "very important" rating, and the four lowest-ranked items are low indeed.

An additional indication of the lack of firmness in the position of eligible nondonors in the general public was noted earlier. On balance, these people were at least slightly supportive of the provision of more rather than less "blood donation recruitment pressure." Our interpretation is that many eligible nondonors would be more comfortable as donors and would not at all mind additional mild intrusions that would push them over the line. Needless to say, the eligible nondonors at the insurance companies were much firmer in their attitudes and were not supportive of additional recruitment pressure.

Eligible nondonors at the insurance companies were far less

Table 7.11 Average importance ratings for nondonation reasons.

	Average rating by		
	Males (n = 55)	Females (n = 86)	All (n = 141)
Nobody asked you personally	1.85	2.08	1.99
No convenient opportunity	2.13	2.22	2.19
Concern with discomfort	2.51	2.48	2.49
Fear of needles	2.66	2.45	2.53
Concern with medical risk	2.67	2.68	2.68
Belief that blood is not really needed	2.76	2.80	2.78

Survey activity: general public.
Population represented: eligible nondonors.
Displayed: average importance rating (very important = 1, fairly important = 2, not important = 3) for each of the given nondonation reasons.

Table 7.12 "Very important" ratings for nondonation reasons.

	Percentage of eligible nondonors who rated given reason "very important"		
	Males (n = 55)	Females (n = 86)	All (n = 141)
Nobody asked you personally	40	37	38
No convenient opportunity	29	28	29
Concern with discomfort	7	20	15
Fear of needles	13	16	14
Concern with medical risk	9	7	8
Belief that blood is not really needed	7	7	7

Survey activity: general public.
Population represented: eligible nondonors.
Note: The three response choices were "very important," "fairly important," and "not important."

likely to provide nondonation reasons such as "Nobody asked me," "Never thought about it," or "No convenient donation opportunity." They were surrounded by solicitation and convenient donation opportunities sufficient to convert into donors many people who would otherwise be nondonors. Remaining an eligible nondonor at the insurance companies may require as conscious a decision as that required to become a donor in a less pervasive blood-collection environment. Tables 7.13–7.15 present data on the insurance companies employees for comparison with tables 7.10–7.12 for the general public. For people who remain eligible nondonors at the insurance companies, fear (of needles, of seeing blood, of having serious donation reactions) replaces the more passive, conjectural nondonation reasons offered by eligible nondonors in the general public.

We believe that most eligible nondonors in the general public responded quite truthfully when providing their reasons for never having given blood. Some were people whom the blood-collection system had not pursued with any intensity. Tables 7.16 and 7.17 provide a comparison of the firmness of nondonor status for eligible nondonors in the general public and in the insurance com-

Table 7.13 Distribution of open-ended reasons for nondonation.

	Percentage of all responses from		
	Males ($n = 15$)	Females ($n = 99$)	All ($n = 114$)
Fear	63	61	61
Other	25	27	27
No convenient opportunity	12	4	5
Never thought about it	0	5	4
Bad previous experience	0	3	3
No real need	0	1	0
Never asked	0	0	0

Survey activity: insurance companies.
Population represented: eligible nondonors.
Displayed: percentage of all open-ended nondonation reasons coded into the given categories.
Notes: For cases in which a respondent provided two reasons, each was given a weight of ½ reason for purposes of this tabulation. Responses to the open-ended request for the respondent's reasons for nondonation are listed for various nondonor groupings in Technical Report 136 of the MIT Operations Research Center.

Table 7.14 Average importance ratings for nondonation reasons.

	Average rating by		
	Males (n = 15)	Females (n = 99)	All (n = 114)
Concern with discomfort	2.13	1.79	1.83
Fear of needles	2.40	1.83	1.91
Concern with medical risk	2.40	2.23	2.25
No convenient opportunity	2.60	2.72	2.70
Belief that blood is not really needed	2.93	2.70	2.73
Nobody asked you personally	2.87	2.86	2.86

Survey activity: insurance companies.
Population represented: eligible nondonors.
Displayed: average importance rating (very important = 1, fairly important = 2, not important = 3) for each of the given nondonation reasons.

Table 7.15 "Very important" ratings for nondonation reasons.

	Percentage of eligible nondonors who rated given reasons "very important"		
	Males (n = 15)	Females (n = 99)	All (n = 114)
Fear of needles	13	46	42
Concern with discomfort	13	43	39
Concern with medical risk	13	24	22
Belief that blood is not really needed	0	10	9
No convenient opportunity	7	7	7
Nobody asked you personally	7	3	4

Survey activity: insurance companies.
Population represented: eligible nondonors.
Note: At the insurance companies, there are very few male nondonors who consider themselves eligible to give blood.

Table 7.16 Firmness of nondonor status, as indicated by agreement with statement "I have made a relatively firm decision not to be a blood donor."

	General public eligible nondonors ($n = 141$)	Insurance companies eligible nondonors ($n = 114$)
Percent agreeing	14	26
Percent not sure	6	48
Percent disagreeing	80	26
Average agreement index	2.67	2.00

Survey activity: general public and insurance companies.
Population represented: eligible nondonors.
Displayed: distribution of responses to and average agreement index (agree = 1, not sure = 2, disagree = 3) for responses to the statement.

Table 7.17 Nondonor average agreement ratings for first-person statements about blood donation.

	Average agreement index	
	General public eligible nondonors ($n = 121$)	Insurance companies eligible nondonors ($n = 84$)
"I would give blood to replace blood used by a friend or relative."	1.07	1.14
"I would give blood if there were an extreme shortage."	1.10	1.33
"A convenient opportunity is all that would be required to get me to give blood once in a while."	1.60	2.28
"I would be more likely to give blood if donors were paid $20 for each donation."	2.80	2.53

Survey activity: general public and insurance companies.
Population represented: eligible nondonors who either disagreed with or were not sure about the statement "I have made a relatively firm decision not to be a blood donor."
Displayed: average agreement index (agree = 1, not sure = 2, disagree = 3) for each of the given statements.

panies. The recruitment system at those companies had converted the less firm nondonors into donors. A further comparison of this type is provided in Table 7.18, which demonstrates that nondonors in the general public made more favorable statements about donation in the future than did the people who had remained nondonors at the insurance companies. The major point is that many eligible nondonors in the general public had not yet had occasion to polarize their blood-donation attitudes one way or the other. People who remained eligible nondonors at the insurance companies, however, had had no shortage of opportunities to remove most elements of conjecture from their attitudes.

Our survey activities also explored how people believed their participation in the whole-blood supply might be affected by a cash payment of $20 (somewhat higher than the typical amount). A large majority of adults believed such payment would be unlikely to increase their own participation, although they did believe many other people would be more willing to give blood in response to such payment.

The data suggest that many eligible nondonors simply have yet to encounter circumstances that force them to think seriously about blood donation. It appears to us that these people are somewhat more lacking in direct solicitation than in being aware of what they consider to be regular, convenient donation opportunities. Reasonably personal forms of solicitation seem likely to convert many of these eligible nondonors into active donors.

Table 7.18 Eligible nondonors' likelihood of donation during next two years.

	General public eligible nondonors ($n = 141$)	Insurance companies eligible nondonors ($n = 114$)
Not likely	46%	62%
Fairly likely	38%	30%
Very likely	16%	8%
Average likelihood index	1.70	1.46

Survey activity: general public and insurance companies.
Population represented: eligible nondonors.
Displayed: distribution of responses to and average likelihood index (not likely = 1, fairly likely = 2, very likely = 3) for responses to the question "All things considered, how likely do you think you are to give blood during the next two years?"

For perspective, it is important to recall that present needs are met easily without a donor base as large as the collection of all eligible potential donors. Whole-blood needs are still far below the level at which we could claim to need some blood from every eligible potential donor.

Attitudes and Reasons of Donors

Along with the misconception that very few people give blood, the literature bursts with the notion that it is terribly important to understand the subtle "reasons" why those rare and unusual people, blood donors, willingly give their blood. Perhaps, the notion continues, we might better foster and propagate these reasons in the general public, or at least better understand how to identify the segments of the public most susceptible to particular types of solicitation.

We have established that, relative to the need, blood donors are many, not few. Furthermore, after extensive experience in asking people why they give blood, we believe pursuit of this issue yields far less information than one might expect. It may be that many donors find an inquiry into their donation reasons to be among the least sensible questions they have heard. Blood donations result from a combination of solicitation, convenient donation opportunity, and the donor's belief that "the need is obvious" and that "there will only be blood if I am willing to give it." For donors who see blood donation as a natural and obvious activity where the value of the gift exceeds the costs of any discomfort associated with it, the pursuit of more detailed reasons for blood donation may be without meaning.

When pushed to provide or select less obvious reasons for their donations, donors' responses are flavored by the reasons supplied to them by their local blood-collection organizations. Sometimes this leads to remarkably inconsistent behavior, such as the common case of people who say they donate blood "to obtain blood coverage for themselves and their associates" but who knowingly give blood much more often than is required to obtain that coverage.

We present some results of our studies with regard to donor "reasons." At the time of our survey research activities, the Houston and New York blood-collection systems were primarily of the individual-responsibility type (actually IR-MC according to the classifications introduced in chapter 2). Responses from these two metropolitan areas are merged in table 7.19 for comparison with responses from people in the Hartford metropolitan area, which is part of a statewide community-responsibility (CR-SG) blood-collection system. Table 7.19 displays average importance ratings from a multiple-choice item about reasons for a donor's most recent blood donation. To make it likely that the respondent could recall the circumstances of his or her most recent blood donation, table 7.19 is limited to responses from people who believed their most recent donation was made within the most recent 3½ years. "Awareness" has the highest average rating from all groups listed in this table. Similar results have been obtained in essentially all our related survey items and with all target populations.

For data such as in table 7.19, we suspect that the high rating of "awareness" represents the good sense of the donors. The relative rankings of other reasons probably result primarily from the publicity and recruiting styles of the blood-collection organizations at the various locations. Table 7.20 provides similar data on people who are unusually active donors relative to common practices in

Table 7.19 Average importance ratings of reasons for most recent donation.

Houston and New York general public ($n = 55$)		Hartford			
		general public ($n = 28$)		insurance companies ($n = 196$)	
Awareness	1.89	Awareness	1.54	Awareness	1.27
Insurance	2.07	Convenience	1.89	Convenience	1.73
Replacement	2.16	Crisis	2.25	Crisis	1.73
Convenience	2.31	Replacement	2.43	Replacement	2.23
Crisis	2.31	Insurance	2.64	Encouragement	2.49
Encouragement	2.47	Encouragement	2.70	Insurance	2.79

Survey activity: general public and insurance companies.
Population represented: donors who gave at least once during the last 3½ years.
Displayed: average importance ratings (very important = 1, fairly important = 2, not important = 3) for each of the following reasons for most recent donation: convenient opportunity, encouragement from someone you know, replacement of blood for a friend or relative, awareness of the normal need of the community for blood, a desire to get some blood insurance so you would receive blood if ever you needed it, and response to a blood-supply crisis. These reasons are abbreviated in the table.

Table 7.20 Average importance ratings for highest-rated reasons for most recent donation by especially active recent donors

Bergen County, N.J. (n = 80)		Hartford (n = 86)		Minneapolis (n = 95)		New York (n = 82)	
Awareness	2.09	Awareness	1.55	Awareness	2.15	Awareness	2.19
Crisis	2.45	Convenience	2.07	Crisis	2.48	Insurance	2.35
Convenience	2.50	Crisis	2.35	Convenience	2.60	Crisis	2.54
Insurance	2.59			Insurance	2.60	Convenience	2.69

Survey activity: frequent and former donors.
Population represented: donors who were unusually active during recent years (selection technique explained in Technical Report 137, MIT Operations Research Center).
Displayed: average importance ratings (especially critical = 1, of considerable importance = 2, relevant but minor = 3, essentially irrelevant = 4) for each of the following reasons for most recent donation: convenience of opportunity, encouragement and/or pressure from associates, replacement of blood for a particular patient, reducing hospital bill for a particular patient, knowledge of a blood-supply crisis, awareness of general need for blood, desire to obtain some form of blood insurance, and curiosity about donation process.
Notes: Of the locations considered here, only Hartford had a community-responsibility (CR-SG) system at the time of our work. Minneapolis had the most distinctly defined of the three individual responsibility systems.
Only reasons with average importance ratings beyond 3 ("relevant but minor") are included in this table.

their localities. (Note that the response scales are slightly different from those used in table 7.19.) The rankings of various "reasons" for donation do, of course, depend on the degree of aggregation of the data. For example, we would expect "encouragement" to be rated as more important by a population composed entirely of first-time donors.

Typical reports in the literature on donor motivation and recruitment describe the reasons provided by donors within one particular blood-collection environment. Not surprisingly, the donors tend to favor those reasons propagated by the local collection organization. The authors of such a study, who usually are involved in one way or another with the local collection organization, typically conclude that the local ideology is in fact the one that gets most donors to give blood.

All our own experiences lead us to believe that participation in the whole-blood supply is the natural, unforced response of a great many people once they are exposed to a mild degree of personal solicitation and some convenient donation opportunities. Almost the entire adult population has been made well aware of the routine need for blood for medical procedures. The blood-collection system reaches out to those populations that are reached easily and that are amenable to fairly efficient collections of blood with low hepatitis infectivity rates. Not surprisingly, members of the pursued populations give a great deal more blood than do members of other population groups. When the unreached people are more carefully solicited, we expect that many of them will also be donors and that their reasons will be no different from those provided by present donors.

Ex-Donors

Professional blood-donor recruiters forever complain about the apparently excessive number of people who used to give blood but who no longer do so. It is generally assumed that their change in behavior results from a conscious decision to cease donating, probably because they have become dissatisfied with the blood-collection organizations. Possible bases for the dissatisfaction are conjectured to be a bad donation experience, news items about the misuse or sale of donated blood, or something else an ex-donor hears or reads about the ills of the collection and distribution system. Each of the two major collection organizations has been known to suggest that it is the other's imperfect practices and performance that have soured the attitudes of so many former donors.

To have a single definition for reference, we use the term *ex-donors* for people who believe their most recent blood donation was made more than about 3½ years before our contact with them.

The existence of a large population of eligible ex-donors should be recognized as an obvious and necessary consequence of such factors as the limited need for blood, the desire to add new people to the donor base, and continuing efforts to draw blood in an efficient manner from the most promising groups.

People become ex-donors for a wide variety of reasons, including changes in real or perceived eligibility (some people in this category later resume donating) and the loss of regular solicitation and/or convenient donation opportunities (often associated with a change of employment or residence). We think it important to consider whether donors become ex-donors primarily as a result of conscious intentions or as an indirect result of externalities.

Tables 7.21 and 7.22 present some basic data about the 53 eligi-

Attitudes and Decisions About Donation

Table 7.21 Comparisons of eligible ex-donors and eligible recent donors.

	Eligible ex-donors (n = 53)	Eligible recent donors (n = 80)
Average age	42	38
Percentage of group that is male	77	60
Average total number of donations	6	14
Average years since most recent donation	8	1
Percentage of group whose most recent donation was made at a hospital	51	29
Percentage of group whose most recent donation was made in present geographic area	60	89
Percentage of group that now has a convenient time and place to give blood regularly	52	84

Survey activity: general public.
Population represented: respondents who had given blood more recently than 1959 and were currently eligible to donate.

Table 7.22 Measures of awareness of ex-donor status.

	Eligible ex-donors (n = 53)	Eligible recent donors (n = 80)
Percentage of group less willing to give again as a result of most recent donation experience	13	5
Percentage of group that had a negative change of attitude toward giving blood since most recent donation	2	3
Percentage of group expecting to make no blood donations in next two years	8	2
Average number of donations group members thought they were likely to make in next two years	2.2	3.1

Survey activity: general public.
Population represented: respondents who had given blood more recently than 1959 and were currently eligible to donate.

ble ex-donors and the 80 eligible "recent donors" (people who gave blood at least once during the most recent 3½ years) from our general-public survey. As the data in these tables indicate, the majority of the eligible ex-donors do not think of themselves as ex-donors. Rather, they are mostly people who now are less connected to some solicitation and donation mechanism than they probably were at an earlier time. Table 7.22 suggests that few eligible ex-donors are troubled or angry about anything related to blood donation. Our interpretation is that most eligible ex-donors will be quite responsive to donation opportunities if and when the blood-collection system finds it desirable to bring them back within its reach.

Comparisons of these data about eligible ex-donors in the general public with data about similar people in the intense blood-collection environment at the insurance companies are interesting. Such comparisons are limited, however, by the not unexpected fact that the blood-related education and solicitation and the donation opportunities at the insurance companies result in an employee population that contains very few eligible ex-donors. In table 7.23 we offer some comparisons of responses from the two

Table 7.23 Donation opportunities and attitudes of ex-donors.

	Eligible ex-donors	
	Insurance companies ($n = 25$)	General public ($n = 53$)
Percentage of group that currently had a convenient time and place to give blood regularly	96	52
Percentage of group less willing to give again as a result of most recent donation experience	48	13
Percentage of group that had had a negative change of attitude toward giving blood since most recent donation	4	2
Percentage of group expecting to make no blood donations in next two years	72	8

Survey activity: general public and insurance companies.
Population represented: eligible respondents whose most recent blood donations were made 3½–16½ years before our survey activities.

sets of eligible ex-donors. As was the case among eligible nondonors, the attitudes of eligible ex-donors at the insurance companies appear to be more strongly formed. As one example of this, note in table 7.23 that 72 percent of the eligible ex-donors at the insurance companies expected to make no blood donations during the next two years. The comparable figure for the eligible ex-donors in the general public was 8 percent. Eligible ex-donors at the insurance companies had consciously selected that status.

In blood banking circles, the one-donation donor is much discussed. It is often contended that there are many ex-donors who have given blood only once and, for whatever reasons, consciously decided to donate no more. Our findings are that most people, if affected at all in motivation by the experience of their initial donation, found the donation easier and more pleasant than they had anticipated and are consequently more willing, rather than less willing, to give again. Our general-public-survey respondents included 53 eligible ex-donors, of whom 18 had made only one donation. Five of these 18 people reported that they were less willing (as opposed to more willing or unchanged in their willingness) to give again, and only one expected to make no donations during the next two years.

Our conclusion is that most eligible ex-donors achieve that status more because of externalities than because of conscious decisions to stop giving blood. Most donors, although surprisingly willing to respond to practical solicitation and donation opportunities, do not go around thinking about blood donation or seeking opportunities to give their blood. Most eligible ex-donors are ex-donors merely because the blood-collection system has found other people, more easily or more efficiently reached, to meet its limited needs.

Intense Collection Environments

We have considered some of the effects of an intense blood-collection environment such as exists at the insurance companies in the Hartford metropolitan area. In such an environment, people who are medically eligible to give blood do so at a much greater rate than do their counterparts in the general public, and eligible nondonors and eligible ex-donors generally enter these categories more consciously and firmly. There are remarkably few eligible ex-donors, especially males, in an intense collection environment.

With a working population that is young, predominantly female, and probably more health-conscious than the general public, the insurance companies provide well over one unit of blood for every two eligible employees per year. Some donors regularly give three or more times each year. A similar average participation level from the entire eligible U.S. population would provide over 40 million units of whole blood per year, more than three times the present annual need.

It is our belief that, even at the insurance companies, most donors are willing to give their blood even more often. Collections at the insurance companies, and elsewhere, are limited by many factors other than the willingness of potential donors. These factors include the limited level of actual blood needs, the subsequent development of reasonable collection goals, and the scaling of collection resources to meet the actual needs. Our primary interest in the blood programs at the insurance companies has been the opportunity they provide for us to learn about public response to blood collection under especially favorable conditions. The fraction of eligible people at the insurance companies who remain nondonors may be relevant to the response of the general public if and when it becomes necessary to extend such thorough solicitation and donation exposure to a larger fraction of the population. At some point such extensions may become impractical and unreasonably expensive. To date, however, we believe that the outreach of the blood-collection organizations has been constrained mainly by their limited need for blood and by the inadequate organization and coordination of some parts of the blood-collection community.

We conclude that the insurance companies provide additional evidence that present and projected blood needs are significantly below any level that would severely test the willingness of the public to give blood under reasonable circumstances.

High School Blood Drives

Our work with high school students provides an opportunity to observe decision-making by young people at a time when many are presented with their first realistic blood solicitation and donation opportunities.

The high school blood programs we studied are watched over by professional staff members of the Red Cross Northeast Regional

Blood Program and appear to be representative of organized high school blood programs. Most of the eligible donors were 17 years old. In Massachusetts and about 25 other states, blood donation at that age requires a signed form expressing parental consent.

A summary of responses to a blood drive by students who did not consider themselves permanently ineligible to give blood appeared in table 7.9. About 26 percent of these students actually donated at what, for many of them, was the first realistic opportunity. An additional 25 percent of the students who did not consider themselves permanently ineligible reported that they tried to participate but had been turned down at home (an especially common situation for females) or judged at least temporarily ineligible by professional personnel at the donation site.

As we did above for the general public and for the insurance companies, we present data on the effect of the first donation experience on students' willingness to give again. We see from table 7.24 that about half of the high school donors believed that their donation experience increased their willingness to give again. About 45 percent of these people believed their donation willingness was not changed, and only about 5 percent said they were less likely to give again because of their initial experience.

The position of the high school nondonors was not particularly firm. Evidence of this appears in tables 7.25 and 7.26. Only about 10 percent of the high school nondonors agreed with the statement "I have made a relatively firm decision not to give blood." A considerably larger fraction of the high school nondonors were "not sure" about the statement than was the case for adult nondonors in the general public. Even students who did not attempt to participate in a high school blood drive reported an average

Table 7.24 Effect of first donation on willingness of high school donors to give again.

	Males ($n = 57$)	Females ($n = 53$)	All ($n = 110$)
"More willing"	40.4%	58.5%	49.1%
"No effect"	52.6%	39.6%	46.4%
"Less willing"	7.0%	1.9%	4.5%

Survey activity: high schools.
Population represented: high school donors.

Table 7.25 Firmness of nondonor status among high school students, as indicated by response to statement "I have made a relatively firm decision not to give blood."

	Male nondonors ($n = 119$)	Female nondonors ($n = 174$)	All nondonors ($n = 293$)
Agreeing	13.4%	6.9%	9.6%
Not sure	37.0%	27.0%	31.1%
Disagreeing	49.6%	66.1%	59.4%

Survey activity: high schools.
Population represented: nondonors 17 years of age or older who did not consider themselves permanently ineligible and believed they had had at least one convenient donation opportunity.

Table 7.26 Intentions of high school students, as indicated by response to the question "Do you think you will try to give blood at your next convenient opportunity?"

Actual and attempted donors			Nondonors		
Males ($n = 81$)	Females ($n = 126$)	All ($n = 207$)	Males ($n = 95$)	Females ($n = 99$)	All ($n = 194$)
1.79	1.54	1.64	2.74	2.54	2.63

Survey activity: high schools.
Population represented: as in table 7.25.
Displayed: average likelihood index ("almost certainly" = 1, "probably" = 2, "maybe, maybe not" = 3, "probably not" = 4, "almost certainly not" = 5) for responses to the question.
Note: "Attempted and actual donors" includes both donors and students who were declared ineligible at the donation site or who were 17 years of age and whose parents would not sign the required permission form.

likelihood on the positive side of "maybe, maybe not" for giving blood at the next convenient opportunity.

For lack of organizational skills on the part of some blood-collection organizations, convenient and well-organized donation opportunities are not provided at some large high schools and some major universities. In other regions, however, 25 percent or more of all blood needs are met by high schools and colleges. Because they encourage participation in the blood supply at a time when people are forming some of their adult behavior patterns, high school and college blood programs are of great importance to the future of the donor base.

Blood Collection Ideology and Policy

Although blood-collection ideology is a prominent topic in discussions and battles between the Red Cross and the American Association of Blood Banks, most citizens have had little opportunity to even become aware of the underlying issues. In our survey activities, strong and consistent attitudes were found only with regard to the purchase of blood from donors. On other ideological issues, such as the relative merits of individual and community responsibility, responses were mild and often inconsistent.

Preferences Among Alternative Collection Organizations

Few people get to make conscious choices among blood-collection organizations. However, using several formats, we asked people whether they would prefer to give their blood to particular collection organizations or to other organizations, or whether they had no preference. Respondents were made aware of all organizations under consideration before they were asked to reply. In the surveys of the general public and the insurance companies, the organizations considered were hospitals, community blood banks, commercial firms that pay donors, and the Red Cross. Average preference ratings for these four types of organizations are shown, by metropolitan area, in table 7.27. Although people tended to prefer the types of organizations that already were the prevalent collectors in their localities, the only strong result was the common disinclination to give blood to a commercial firm that pays for it. If separate versions of the data in table 7.27 are prepared for donors and for eligible nondonors, the results are quite similar (with the one exception that nondonors rate hospitals slightly higher than

Table 7.27 Preferences among types of blood-collection organizations.

	Average preference ratings			
	Hartford ($n = 119$)	Houston ($n = 92$)	New York ($n = 116$)	All ($n = 327$)
Hospital	0.17	0.32	0.21	0.22
Community blood bank	0.09	0.37	0.14	0.19
Commercial firm that pays donors	−0.78	−0.70	−0.79	−0.76
Red Cross	0.38	0.00	0.09	0.17

Survey activity: general public.
Population represented: donors and eligible nondonors.
Displayed: average preference ratings ("prefer" = 1, "no difference" = 0, "rather another organization" = −1) for given types of blood-collection organizations.

do donors, probably because nondonors are more likely to assume that hospitals are the usual places for blood donation). People were favorably inclined toward all actual and potential blood-collection agencies (including public hospitals, private hospitals, and the Salvation Army), with the exception of commercial firms that purchase blood.

We did not attempt to estimate psychological profiles for survey respondents. However, from the demographic and other information we have from all our survey activities, we see no reason to believe that the major primary blood-collection organizations and ideologies attract significantly different types of people.

Attitudes Toward Payment for Whole-Blood Donations

Whether the question is put in terms of their own whole-blood donations or in terms of donations made by others, a large majority of our respondents had a very negative attitude toward the purchase of blood from donors. One manifestation of this was seen in table 7.27. Even eligible nondonors, including those who considered themselves firm nondonors, were not sympathetic to having their communities meet blood needs by purchasing blood.

It is interesting to ask whether such feelings are predicated more on ideological or on practical grounds. Although our results are not conclusive, they suggest that the negative feelings about the purchase of blood are based more on ideology than on beliefs about the medical consequences. There were significantly more people opposed to the purchase of blood donations that there were people who believed the quality of the blood supply would be decreased by it.

Except for male nondonors at the high schools, all our survey populations disagreed firmly with the statement "I would be much more likely to give blood if donors were paid $20 for each donation." Of the 132 eligible nondonors in the general-public survey, 88 percent disagreed with the statement, 2 percent were not sure, and only 10 percent agreed. However, a clear majority of all populations surveyed believed that a $20 payment would make many other people willing to donate. The consistency of this result among different sets of respondents is displayed in table 7.28.

Many people, including those opposed to the purchase of blood from donors and unlikely to find additional motivation for donation if offered payment for their own blood, do respect the right of other persons to sell their blood. Some of our pretest surveys included an item about attitudes toward legislation to outlaw the

Table 7.28 Responses to statement "If all blood donors were paid $20 for each donation, many more people would be willing to be blood donors."

	n	Percentage of people whose response was			Average agreement index
		"Agree"	"Not sure"	"Disagree"	
High school nondonors	188	79	14	7	1.3
High school actual and attempted donors	209	74	19	7	1.3
General public eligible nondonors	151	71	4	25	1.5
Insurance company donors	273	57	22	21	1.6
Insurance company eligible nondonors	124	60	16	24	1.7
General public donors	200	58	7	35	1.8

Survey activity: general public, insurance companies, and high schools.
Population represented: as indicated in table.
Displayed: distribution of responses to and average agreement index ("agree" = 1, "not sure" = 2, "disagree" = 3) for responses to the statement.

purchase of blood donations, and the overall response was essentially neutral.

Individual and Community Responsibility

With the exception of monetary payment, people are generally supportive of all reasonable arrangements for meeting whole-blood needs. Only at the insurance companies, where people receive large amounts of blood-related information and large doses of the community-responsibility point of view, did we find a majority of our survey respondents in disagreement with the statement "Patients and their families should be expected to arrange for replacing blood they receive." Even in the Hartford metropolitan area, in a state with one of the oldest operating community-responsibility collection systems in the United States, a slight majority of the actual and attempted blood donors in the general-public survey agreed with the statement. Responses to this item by several populations appear in table 7.29.

Although almost all populations displayed majority support for the individual-responsibility concept of blood replacement, they also displayed similar support for community responsibility. Table 7.30 shows results for a survey item concerned with prefer-

Table 7.29 Attitudes toward blood replacement, as indicated by responses to the statement "Patients and their families should be expected to arrange for replacing blood they receive."

	n	Percentage of people whose response was			Average agreement index
		"Agree"	"Not sure"	"Disagree"	
General public					
Hartford	164	51	9	40	1.89
Houston	132	72	4	24	1.52
New York	162	75	5	20	1.46
All	458	65	6	29	1.63
Insurance companies					
All	503	26	23	51	2.26

Survey activity: general public and insurance companies.
Population represented: all respondents.
Displayed: distribution of and average agreement index ("agree" = 1, "not sure" = 2, "disagree" = 3) for responses to the statement.

Table 7.30 Preferred source for most blood needs, as indicated by responses to the question "From which group do you think your area should get most of the blood needed—from paid donors, family associates of patients, or people who give blood to the entire community?"

		Percentage of people in group preferring		
	n	Paid donors	Family and associates	Community donors
Houston and New York general public				
Eligible nondonors	86	7	34	59
Donors	115	1	32	67
Hartford general public				
Eligible nondonors	50	0	14	86
Donors	66	2	4	94
Insurance companies				
Eligible nondonors	115	2	22	76
Donors	258	1	13	86

Survey activity: general public and insurance companies.

ences between individual-responsibility and community-responsibility systems as the sources of most of a community's blood supply. The effect of the long-established community-responsibility practices in Connecticut can be seen in this table.

Most people have not formed consistent attitudes on community and individual responsibility. Because donors are likely to know more about this than nondonors, we present some data for the donors in our general-public survey work. Even of the 115 donors who agreed that patients and their families should be expected to arrange for blood replacement, 70 percent preferred donors who give their blood to the entire community to be the primary source of the blood supply. (The other choices were paid donors and replacement donors.) Similarly, about 60 percent of the 138 donors who preferred a blood supply obtained from people who give blood to the entire community also agreed that patients and their families should be expected to replace blood.

Although differences between community- and individual-responsibility systems may have significant impact on the situation of a patient who has received blood, we see little reason to suspect that the issue seriously affects donation behavior.

Conclusions

Because of what they hear directly and indirectly from the blood-collection organizations and because they are quite likely to be aware of at least one personal acquaintance who has received a blood transfusion, people are well aware of the routine need for whole-blood donations. Opportunities to donate blood and public participation in the whole-blood supply are broadly distributed.

About half the people who consider themselves eligible to give blood, as well as many people who are not now eligible, have given blood at least once. The actual number of donors in any particular year (now about 8 million) is a consequence of the limited need for blood rather than of public resistance to blood donation. Highly organized blood-collection environments can produce, apparently without great personal strain or financial expense, per capita blood collections far in excess of average national needs. The dominant "reason" for blood donations is simply a general awareness of the continuing need for blood. Mobilization of potential donors does, of course, require a reasonable degree of organizational support in terms of personal solicitation chains and donation convenience.

Many "ex-donors" have simply lost some of the solicitation and donation opportunity to which they were formerly exposed. Only a small number of the eligible ex-donors have made conscious decisions to withdraw from the blood supply. Any reasonable blood program with a broad donor base must have a large population of donors who have not given blood during the most recent few years.

Most people who consider themselves eligible to give blood but who have never done so are not firm in their status as nondonors. Many are people whom the blood collection system has not yet pursued much. Many are in favor of, rather than opposed to, additional recruitment pressure.

Few people are comfortable with the notion of obtaining whole blood by paying donors. As far as we can tell, the issue of community versus individual responsibility is of little interest to the public, either as a matter of ideology or as a determinant of willingness to give blood.

Public attitudes and unwillingness to give are not the primary causes of the limited difficulties the blood collection and distribution system still experiences. As is clear from discussions in earlier chapters, we think the whole-blood supply performs surprisingly well. Although intensified public education about blood needs may have several benefits, it certainly does not appear necessary for the achievement of an adequate blood supply. Professionalization and coordination of the collection organizations seem to us the more critical issues. The public is more than willing to do its share.

8 Cross-National Comparisons

The most interesting aspect of blood banking to compare cross-nationally is the social organization of blood collections. There are, to be sure, cross-national variations in the medical practices associated with blood banking, but these variations are usually minor in their impact and are almost always attributable to obvious differences in national wealth. If the British long persisted in the use of glass bottles instead of plastic bags for collecting blood, it was not because their physicians preferred glass to plastic containers but rather because Great Britain could not afford to switch to plastic as quickly as some countries.[1] Medical innovations tend to move freely across political boundaries, hindered mainly by economics. In contrast, the persistent variations in social organization apparently are due to national preferences, and therefore are more difficult to explain. The Danes and the Swedes, for example, pay blood donors, but quite differently. In Denmark the payment goes to donor organizations and is used collectively for cultural activities such as the group purchase of tickets to concerts and ballets, whereas payments to Swedish donors are made and spent individually.

The desire, of course, is for simple explanations for the variations in social organization that are observed; the corresponding danger is that the explanations will be simplistic. According to Titmuss's *The Gift Relationship*, because the United States allows blood to be bought and sold it suffers from unnecessary shortages, unconscionable waste, and avoidable illness and death caused by transfusion-induced hepatitis. The profit motive leads donors and procurers of blood to lie about the quality of their product, thus endangering the health of recipients. Great Britain, by contrast, supposedly suffers none of these problems because its government plans centrally the procurement of blood and does not pay for donations.

However, Titmuss, in his eagerness to find fault with the market system, was inaccurate in his description and analysis. Commercial blood (blood bought and sold for private profit) made up a declining share of blood collections in the United States when Titmuss wrote. As we said, American blood banking has always been dominated by nonprofit organizations. Thus, Titmuss was largely attacking a straw man, devastating as that attack may have been. Moreover, central planning and voluntarism in blood banking, which Titmuss favored, do not guarantee improved performance. Waste and shortages exist in both the United States and Great Britain. The most inclusive national survey of blood banking in the United States was done by Booz Allen Hamilton, Inc., under the sponsorship of the National Heart and Lung Institute.[2] This survey reported the "outdating" rate for blood as 12.9 percent of 1971 collections, a figure quite close to the rate of 11.8 percent for the same year reported by the British Transfusion Service to the Council of Europe's Public Health Committee.[3] Other surveys report that blood is often in short supply, not only in Newark but also in South London, and that donors are either reluctant to give or inadequately solicited during vacation periods and holidays in both Great Britain and the United States.[4]

Titmuss's most serious charge was that the American system promotes needless death and ill health. A trade in blood, Titmuss argued, creates incentives for socially irresponsible and medically dangerous behavior. When there is a market in blood, derelicts, drug addicts, and others with both a high risk of being hepatitis carriers and a need for money have an interest in concealing their poor health. Those who pay them and resell their blood have the same interest. In the United States, where some blood is still exchanged for money, transfusion-induced hepatitis is an important medical problem. (Although precise figures are not available, estimates range from 1,000 to 3,700 deaths and 90,000 to 120,000 hospitalizations each year—an infection rate of approximately 4 cases per 100 transfusions). In Great Britain, where a cup of tea or a glass of stout is about all one can get for a blood donation, transfusion-induced hepatitis is considered rare, with perhaps a seventh of the American rate. Money, it would seem, is the root of at least one evil.

However, the control of transfusion-induced hepatitis is more complicated that Titmuss would have us believe. As we noted in chapter 4, not all paid-for blood is commercially acquired blood and not all volunteer blood is safe. Some of our leading medical institutions (the Mayo Clinic and Massachusetts General Hospital, for example) have at times paid some of their blood donors and have had lower rates of transfusion-induced hepatitis than has been the experience with volunteer blood in their areas. Much depends on the care with which donors are screened. Race and ethnicity also seem to be important correlates of the risk of hepatitis infection. Orientals apparently have higher carrier rates than whites. Among whites, those of Southern European origin have higher rates than do those of Northern European origin.

These relationships help explain the variation in national transfusion-hepatitis rates. Sweden, which pays all of its blood donors, has a very low rate. Japan, which switched from a largely paid donor system to an essentially all-volunteer system in the mid-1960s, still has a very high rate.[5] The low rate in Britain relative to the United States is probably due more to the fact that British blood is being used than to the fact that all British donors are volunteers. The National Transfusion Service, the government agency that manages the blood system in Great Britain, apparently agrees, for it discreetly discriminates against new immigrants in its collection procedures. Regional units of the Transfusion Service avoid scheduling collection visits at factories and other sites where there are large concentrations of Pakistanis, Indians, Jamaicans, or other immigrant groups. Blood collected from donors born in Asian, African, and Caribbean countries (and certain other countries, but not the United States) is labeled as high in hepatitis risk (in code) and is then not used, if possible, for direct transfusion. A very rational policy perhaps, but not one that the British advertise, not one reported by Titmuss, and not one that most Americans would endorse.

Comparing the social organization of blood banking throughout the world is a difficult task, and not only because of the paucity of data (a common problem in comparative analyses). As we will note, the data that exist are not always reliable. In the case of blood donations, it seems, governments and blood-collection agencies as well as individuals have incentive to lie or, at best, report only the most favorable truths.

The Preference for "Volunteers"

Every international organization active in blood-banking affairs has taken a stand against compensation for blood donations. The League of Red Cross Societies (officially, the International Federation of National Red Cross, Red Crescent, and Red Lion and Sun Societies), representing member organizations in 122 countries, condemns payments for blood.[6] The World Health Organization, a unit of the United Nations, opposes paid donations.[7] The Public Health Committee of the Council of Europe recommends against the use of nonvolunteer donors,[8] as does the International Society of Blood Transfusion[9] (the international professional organization in transfusion matters), the International Federation of Blood Donor Associations,[10] and the World Federation of Hemophilia (ref. 10). The objection they all raise to nonvolunteer donors is clearly more moral than medical. Hepatitis, it is admitted, is not a significant problem in most developed countries, because of their affluence and their population characteristics. And although many underdeveloped countries have high rates of transfusion-induced hepatitis, their other health problems necessarily dwarf its local importance. Many more people die because of malnutrition and poor sanitation in these countries than because of transfusion hepatitis. The concern, rather, is with the tainting of a blood donation. In order to be worthy, the gift of life is thought to require a nonmaterialistic motive.

One cannot avoid noticing, however, that there is great ambiguity in the definitions of "voluntary donation" that are offered. A voluntary donation is one given "without coercion," all would agree.[11] But is not social pressure such as that generated by patriotic, religious, and organizationally based appeals coercive? It is precisely this type of pressure that some, including the Red Cross, think is most effective in stimulating additional blood donations.[12] A hungry man might feel compelled to donate, but so too might a hounded man. Which one is less coerced? Flags, religious symbols, and currency are all at times used to manipulate people.

It is also often suggested that "any reward, service or allowance received by the donor must not be such that it acts in itself as the incentive to give blood" (ref. 11). Does that mean that there should be no reward for donations? It is not clear. Nearly all blood banks offer cookies or sandwiches and tea or orange juice to their donors, but these gifts are only meant to replenish nutrients. The People's Republic of China, however, offers its blood donors a cash "nutritional supplement" that is the equivalent of a half a month's earnings for a rural worker.[13] Too much replenishment?

Many blood-collection systems provide compensation for travel costs donors incur in reaching and returning from a donation center, obviously justified expenditures that are not in themselves inducements to give. But what about compensated time off from work or extra days of vacation provided donors? Iranian soldiers once routinely received ten days' leave for blood donation—a tempting offer to homesick recruits, one might think.[14] Until the recent financial crisis, New York City policemen received two days off at full pay for a voluntary blood donation. Given a policeman's wage in New York, the "non-inducing" reward for a pint of their blood was approximately $150.[15]

Obviously, there is room for much interpretation in the identification of the altruistic donor. As one acute observer has commented, agreements on the definition of voluntarism in blood donation are as difficult to achieve as agreements on the definition of amateurism for international athletic competitions.[16] The ambiguity, though, is not without function, for in its absence very few nations or blood-collection agencies could claim a total or near-total reliance on volunteer donations. Canada, Great Britain, France, Switzerland, and the Netherlands do not pay donors but surely do not lack in mechanisms for applying social pressures on prospective donors. Red Cross strictures notwithstanding, certain Red Cross affiliates (the Greek Society, for instance) provide cash awards to donors, claiming a national shortage of blood. And almost everywhere there are offers of paid days off or compensation for time lost from work for the "voluntary" donor.

The real embarrassment, of course, is to offer money directly for blood. Money changing hands for blood evokes the wrong moral image, making crass what for many must always be an act of altruistic love. It matters not, apparently, that blood banks conduct transactions with each other and with hospitals in the same currency and that days off from work have a cash equivalency. Blood donors, in this view, simply should not be allowed to appear to be of impure motive.

Surprisingly, money payments for blood donations are more the practice in communist societies than they are in capitalist societies. The Soviet Union pays some of its donors, as do most of the East European countries and the People's Republic of China. Communist abhorrence of markets, it would seem, is not absolute. Perhaps this is the result of the antagonism between voluntarism and the state inherent in such societies. "A task worth doing is a task work compensating" may be the citizen's protective credo under communism. It is the state, not the individual, that decides what tasks are worth doing in a communist society. The state then must provide the appropriate incentive. For at least some in these societies, this means that monetary or monetarily convertible rewards are demanded before the task is accomplished. There are neither private charities nor pools of charitable labor under communism.

Or perhaps this surprising reliance on financial incentives has to do with the relatively low stage of economic development of the communist nations. Cash payments for blood donations are common in the Third World, where most people have to worry too much about their own economic survival to afford to be charitable. Communist poverty, egalitarian though it may be, also may limit the exercise of altruistic urges.

Soviet policy is to eliminate the reliance on paid donors for routine blood resource needs, and the claim is that the percentage of volunteer donors is increasing.[17] Well it might be. Volunteer donors in the Soviet Union receive an extra vacation day and preferential access to resorts in addition to the customary two days off (one to give blood and the other to recuperate) and two free meals afforded all Soviet donors, paid or not. The cash value of the extra vacation day and the opportunity to sun oneself on the Black Sea beach likely exceed the remuneration provided paid donors. The advantage is, however, that cash is not directly paid, thus increasing the voluntary portion of the collections.[18]

Capitalist societies also are embarrassed by a reliance on paid donors. American health agencies, encouraged by the Red Cross, are seeking the elimination of all paid whole-blood donations, nonprofit collections as well as commercial collections. To discourage its use, paid-for blood in the United States must now be labeled as such. Blood given in exchange for a day off or to ensure its availability, though, is not considered to have been given for a cash reward and thus counts as a voluntary contribution in official statistics.[19]

The Japanese managed a rapid switch from a near total dependence on paid blood to an almost entirely voluntary blood system in the mid-1960s. The precipitating event apparently was the contraction of hepatitis from commercially procured blood by the American ambassador, who was hospitalized for stab wounds received in an assassination attempt. This exercise in collective guilt, however, has been somewhat futile because of the endemic nature of hepatitis in the Japanese people. Positive hepatitis B antigen test rates in Japan for volunteer blood are 20 times those for Red Cross blood in the United States.[20]

Only the Swedes remain steadfast in official adherence to a policy of donor payments. A proposal by Swedish medical authorities to adopt a Danish-style collective reward system for blood donations, with the money to be earmarked for charity, was recently rejected. It seems that the Swedish blood-donation payments, modest though they might be, are untaxed, and that this benefit was too great for the heavily taxed Swedes to give up.

Organizational Variations

Blood banking is organized differently in nearly every nation. The structure of the medical system, the relationship between public and private organizations in the society, and unique historical events appear to produce the variations. If there is a universal tendency, it is toward assigning one organization exclusive authority to collect and provide blood within a defined territory. This tendency is at times resisted by hospitals out of fear of dependence on a monopolistic supplier of a vital resource.

The British have organized blood banking as a specialized component of their National Health Service, the governmental provider of health services. The Transfusion Service, structured to parallel the regional organization of the National Health Service, staffs a blood center to supply the needs of each health-service region. Most large British hospitals, however, maintain panels of blood donors that are separate from those maintained by the Transfusion Service. In London the British Red Cross operates a donor service to provide hospitals with fresh whole blood, a product that some practitioners prefer to use for special cases although the Transfusion Service is said to find it both inconvenient to supply and medically unnecessary. Although the amount of blood obtained from the alternative sources is not large relative to the collections of the Transfusion Service, the existence of the alternative source of supply gives an indication that British hospitals are unwilling to commit themselves completely to the preferences of a single supplier, even one that is (like most of the hospitals themselves) an arm of the National Health Service.

In Sweden, it is difficult for the government to permit private organizations to share medical service functions, because the demarcation between public and private activities is nearly absolute. In the United States, private organizations are allowed to compete for the control of medical functions that are elsewhere largely governmental. And in the Netherlands and Switzerland, the governments can easily assign a medical function exclusively to a single private organization and expect no controversy. Thus, blood-collection organizations, the Red Cross included, must adjust to the local opportunities afforded them.

Red Cross–affiliated societies are active in over 120 nations. As is the case with the American National Red Cross, the various Red Cross societies seek a role in blood collections both for the humanitarian purpose of providing blood to the ill and the injured and in order to enhance their other social-welfare programs through the generation of favorable publicity. In 58 countries the Red Cross is permitted to participate directly in blood-collection activities, although in only 13 (Australia, Belgium, Canada, Cuba, Finland, Indonesia, Japan, the Netherlands, Nicaragua, the Philippines, South Korea, Switzerland, and Thailand) is this role exclusive. In the remaining 60-plus nations the Red Cross is relegated to donor recruitment and blood-donation promotion or is totally excluded from involvement in blood procurement.[21]

Idiosyncratic reasons govern the structure and character of the Red Cross national programs. In Denmark, the scouting organization thought of blood collections first. In the United States, the Red Cross must share blood-banking responsibilities with hospitals and free-standing blood centers, largely because of the structure of the blood program during World War II. And the Red Cross is totally absent from Israel, preferring instead an international affiliation with the Red Crescent Societies that are active in the Arab nations.

Trading in Blood

Irrespective of who is in charge, many national blood programs have recently been placed under increasing strain. The common practice in most nations has been to derive plasma resources from whole-blood collections, integrating both functions in a single blood-banking system. Advances in fractionation and therapy, however, have dramatically raised the demand for plasma products. Many programs therefore face the dilemma of either significantly increasing their whole-blood collections, paying their own plasmapheresis donors, or participating directly in the international market for blood fractions. Because modern medical facilities generate a growing demand for the fractions, this dilemma has been particularly acute for the developed nations.

However, the United States, which reduced its dependence on commercial whole-blood collections at just about the time when the important plasma technical advances were being made, has been largely immune from the problem. American commercial blood collectors did not withdraw entirely from the blood business, but rather concentrated their efforts on plasmapheresis collections for pharmaceutical companies preparing plasma products. Relying on paid plasma donors, the production of blood fractions in the United States stands apart from the whole-blood collection system and has kept pace well with rising therapeutic demands.

In contrast, the West European nations and Japan, which usually fractionate plasma from blood units donated as part of their whole-blood procurement system, have experienced shortages. Many of these nations have long been among the adamant resisters to the participation of commercial collectors in blood procurement. They are experiencing supply problems now because their blood-system managers have not invested sufficient resources in plasma collection and plasma-derivative-manufacturing facilities to keep up with the demand for plasma products (apparently believing that other health needs deserve higher budget priorities), and because a reliance for plasma on voluntary whole-blood collections often results in either shortages of donors or collections of excess red cells.

The Europeans have attempted to cope with the problem in a variety of ways. They have sought to persuade physicians to use packed cells instead of whole blood so as to increase the supply of available plasma,[22] they have attempted to negotiate exchanges between surplus and short areas,[23] and they have promoted increased whole-blood donations in order to gain sufficient quantities of plasma for fractionation.[24] A few of these efforts have succeeded. Sweden pays a higher fee for pheresis donors and purchases plasma when needed from Finland and Ireland. Belgium, Switzerland, and West Germany, which have sufficient whole-blood supplies, exchange their surplus red cells for blood-collection supplies (plastic bags, transfusion kits, and the like) with the Greater New York Blood Program, which still experiences shortages of unpaid blood donors but is determined to avoid commercial suppliers even if it means obtaining red cells in Europe.[25] But more often than not there have been either embarrassing surpluses of red cells or shortages of blood fractions. Inevitably there has been some resort to the international plasma-product market.

As mentioned in chapter 6, the extent of the market is difficult to determine precisely. The trade is managed by large American, Japanese, and European pharmaceutical firms, who along with their purchasers and suppliers have historically preferred secrecy to public disclosure. Most of the plasma in international transactions is obtained through brokers, and at least some of it (though less than previously believed) is thought to originate in Third World nations. The fear on the part of the World Health Organization has been that "blood farming" activities are being created in which a corps of professional donors in poor countries provide plasma, to the detriment of their own health, in order to support themselves and their families. Few governments in the Third World have admitted to permitting such an arrangement to operate in their nations, but it is thought that the way has been paved through official corruption as well as the gift of needed medical equipment and supplies for the local health system. Little is known about the care and screening of donors or fees they receive, though the belief is that it is all quite meager.[26] Though there is less concern about this now than previously, much international anguish still exists over the trade in blood between the poor countries and the richest. An effort is being made to ban the trade, but this is likely to occur only when the prime consuming nations, including the European countries, are self-sufficient in the production of plasma derivatives. Table 8.1 shows the current dependence on imported blood products.

Ironically, it may be American donors whose health is at risk, as the United States is now thought to be the major source of blood for the international market. Instead of the trade in blood being between the poor countries and the richest, it may be largely between the United States and other countries, rich or poor. The United States alone in the world possesses a significant surplus of plasma and the production capacity to convert it into commercial products for export. In recognition of this fact, European and Japanese pharmaceutical firms are expanding their investment in the United States to retain a share of the market.

Table 8.1 Estimated imports of blood products in selected countries (percentage of value of current consumption).

Netherlands	11
Belgium	36
Switzerland	40
Britain	50
Denmark	52
Norway	68
Japan	98

Source: International Federation of Pharmaceutical Manufacturers Association, cited in "America the Blood Bank," *Economist*, October 17, 1981, p. 87.

An Unjaundiced View

The outline of ideologies presented in chapter 2 provides a framework for summarizing the international situation in blood banking. We distinguished between individual responsibility and community responsibility in the provision of blood for medical use, and between the designation of blood as a special good or a market commodity in its acquisition. The ideal blood-banking system, the one toward which all nations claim to strive, involves blood being considered both a community responsibility and a special good. Under this scheme no one is required to provide for his own blood needs and no one is paid for a donation. In practice, however, most developed nations maintain a system in which blood is a community responsibility and a market commodity.

The United States stands alone among developed nations in having significant elements of its blood-banking system asserting that the provision of blood is an individual responsibility. This operating ideology is rapidly diminishing in importance and has little practical consequence for individuals in time of need. Still, its existence isolates the United States among national blood-banking programs and causes much foreign puzzlement. Titmuss was but one of many who have wondered whether the notion that an individual should be held responsible for the blood he needs to survive a medical crisis does not take the philosophy of American individualism beyond the limits of reason.

But if Americans appear hard-hearted, Europeans and others appear dishonest. The United States openly permits a market in blood. Almost everywhere else it is denied. And yet, in most nations blood remains a market commodity, denials notwithstanding. The incentives provided donors belie their official voluntary status. Although money does not pass hands in the blood bank, vacation days and meals are money in another form or at another time. Worse still from this perspective is the practice of buying plasma products in the world market (and thus largely from the United States). The products obtained invariably are manufactured from purchased plasma. The moral stain of directly paying the donors is avoided, but only by dealing in blood through intermediaries.

The few nations that remain true to the belief that blood deserves special reverence are also not without fault. Switzerland, the United Kingdom, and a handful of others seek to be free of the supposed immorality of paying blood donors, directly or indirectly. To do so, however, they either must overbleed their citizens to obtain sufficient supplies of plasma or deny them vital plasma products.[27] What price purity?

Only the underdeveloped countries deserve sympathy. There hepatitis is rampant and blood scarce. Paid for or not, donation remains dangerous. Even when supplies are sufficient and obtained with communal charity, it is too often not the gift of life.

9 Blood Policy

There is a sense of unease surrounding every discussion of blood policy. Some people faint at the sight of blood or even its mention. Others expect a seamy tale to unfold. They anticipate being told that a significant portion of the blood supply is collected from destitute alcoholics who line up in the morning at storefronts to give their diseased blood in exchange for the money to buy their next bottle. They are certain that there will be mention of chronic shortages, unconscionable waste, and much illness and death due to the transfusion of tainted blood. They believe, but do not really want to know, that the poor and the helpless are exploited by evil people who profit greatly from a trade in blood.

In fact, the American blood system is much better than this vision. The shortages that occur are few, temporary, and relatively easily corrected. Middle-class donors abound. Hardly anyone is paid cash for their red cells. The quality of the blood supply is high and carefully monitored. Little disease is transmitted by transfusions, and that which is is largely unavoidable. Nonprofit agencies manage the bulk of blood collections and do so with great efficacy and dedication.

Even so, the sense of unease is understandable. In part it is cultivated and in part it reflects historic fact. In their never-ending quest to secure donors, some blood-collection agencies have resorted to exaggerated advertising that encourages the public to believe that the supply of blood is always precarious. The implication of their appeals is that, without immediate response by every potential donor, the supply of safe blood cannot be assured to those who may be in desperate need. As blood is the fluid of life, high drama is easily achieved in the messages.

Most collection agencies exercise restraint in advertising for blood donors, offering quiet, rational appeals instead of emotional ones. Nevertheless, it is difficult for them to avoid completely the hint of impending disaster. The many amateur recruiters aiding their efforts are difficult to control. Moreover, collectors see little advantage in lulling the public into complacency about the need for blood donations. It is better for them to keep the public slightly on edge about the availability of safe blood.

To be sure, during the forty years in which transfusions have become a common medical therapy there have been areas in the United States that have experienced important deficiencies in their blood collections. Unscrupulous collectors have exploited these situations and the fear that they would develop elsewhere in order to draw blood wherever it was convenient, including the skid rows that exist in many cities. Ignorance or indifference about the dangers of hepatitis transmission permitted the use of unsafe blood they gathered. Although this type of blood collection has essentially disappeared in the United States, its image persists. What the public does not generally know is that blood for human use may now only be drawn by licensed facilities, that federal regulations govern the safety of the blood supply, that effective tests for certain strains of hepatitis are routinely applied, and that nearly all whole-blood donations are made without monetary reward.

Just as the public is misinformed about the blood system, so too is much of the public debate about blood policy. The driving forces behind the improvements in blood safety and supply have been scientific and organizational advances. The development of hepatitis-detection techniques by medical researchers has reduced but not yet eliminated the threat of disease transmission through blood transfusion. The recognition of the value of blood-component therapy by physicians has expanded the availability of blood supplies, as has the use of improved preservation methods. The perfection of pheresis techniques has permitted the large-scale collection of plasma to meet the growing demand for fractions. The professionalization of blood collection has improved the supply. So has the involvement of major drug firms in the production of plasma products. The debate over blood policy, however, has centered on the morality of a market for blood.

The Underlying Issue

Paid blood donation developed in the United States because of the inadequacies of the voluntary collection effort. The failure of the Red Cross to establish its desired monopoly because of internal problems and the hostility that exists toward the organization in some regions created shortfalls in voluntary collections. Nonprofit community blood centers and local hospitals filled the gaps, but not completely. In contrast with the case in many other countries, the U.S. government did not ban the commercial collection of blood. Entrepreneurs, some scrupulous and some not, saw an opportunity to make money serving the rising demand for blood and established their own collection facilities. Physicians ordering blood for their patients were concerned primarily with a sure supply, not with its source. The postponement of operations because of inadequate availability of blood means lost surgical fees and patients placed in jeopardy. Hospitals, as the ordering agents for blood, responded to the demands of physicians and the needs of patients by favoring whatever collection mechanism seemed to guarantee the continuous local availability of blood. Compared with the urgency of having blood when needed, the ideology of the collection agent and sources of the blood seemed irrelevant or at best of secondary interest.

Gradually, the nonprofit blood collection agencies improved their operations. The Red Cross overcame some of its internal management problems and, along with the community blood banks, professionalized donor recruitment and blood-bank management. The recognition that reliable supplies were of great concern to hospitals spurred the development of interbank exchanges and better inventory-control techniques by the nonprofit collectors.

Hepatitis became an issue only in the 1960s, when the awareness of the disease began to rise. Until then, neither the commercial nor the nonprofit collectors devoted much effort to its detection in the blood supply. The fact that paid donors obtained through storefront operations were more likely to be carriers of the disease was used by some nonprofit collectors to enhance their competitive position. Attempts were made, sometimes successfully, to institute state labeling requirements that would identify commercially collected blood, with the implication that it was unsafe to transfuse. This occurred even though some nonprofit collectors had relatively high hepatitis carrier rates among their donors as well. Hepatitis control thus became a device by which the nonprofit sector of blood banking sought to improve blood safety and to eliminate competition from commercial rivals.

Discussions of hepatitis-control techniques quickly broaden into a debate over the morality of money exchanges for blood donations. It was argued that money exchanges were a corrupting force in blood collections, causing donors and blood bankers to conceal the poor quality of their product and thus threatening the lives of those in need of blood. Donations, some believed, should only be made for altruistic motives in order to strengthen the bonds of community. Economists rushed to defend the market from this collectivistic attack. If permitted to operate freely, they argued, the market could distinguish by price various qualities of blood and could effectively match demand with supply.

The debate, despite its moments of eloquence, was of little consequence in terms of its effect on the structure of blood banking in the United States or the incidence of hepatitis. Except in a few urban areas (for example Miami, Chicago, and Los Angeles), paid blood donations had never been more than a supplement to the overall blood supply during the last 20 years. The commercial collectors were by the early 1970s deeply involved in the rapidly growing plasma market. Several had been acquired by the major drug firms producing blood derivatives, while others had become the drug firms' contract suppliers of plasma.

However, government attention was attracted by the debate. Some officials in the Department of Health, Education, and Welfare found in the link between hepatitis and paid blood donations justification for another attempt to realign the organization of blood banking in the United States. At their initiative, a National Blood Policy was promulgated that included the following goal:

To encourage, foster, and support efforts to bring into being an all-voluntary blood donation system and to eliminate commercialism in the acquisition of whole blood and blood components for transfusion purposes. The ultimate aims of this policy are improvement in the quality of the supply of blood and blood products and the development of an appropriate ethical climate for the increasing use of human tissues for therapeutic medical purposes. In this context, the term commercialism applies to the relationship between the donor and the blood bank and focuses primarily on those commercial relationships which have encouraged reliance on blood from sectors of society in which transmissible hepatitis is particularly prevalent . . . .

The policy was to be implemented by private action, although resort to legislation if necessary was threatened.

Its phraseology notwithstanding, the National Blood Policy was intended neither as a hepatitis-control measure nor as a direct assault on commercialism in blood banking. The criteria for monitoring its implementation included no goal for the reduction of hepatitis. Plasma collection was explicitly excluded from early reorganization. Instead, attention was directed toward such problems as the regionalization of blood banking and the use of replacement fees, which had been the traditional obstacles to the amalgamation of the major nonprofit blood collectors. The government was initiating the third effort at reconciliation between the Red Cross and the AABB. Cartelization was the intent.

The American Blood Commission

In 1974 the American Blood Commission was founded to implement the National Blood Policy. Unlike previous attempts to bring together the feuding elements of the blood-banking community, the Commission included in its membership donor and consumer organizations as well as blood-collection agencies and other organizations directly involved in the delivery and financing of health-care services. Among the professional affiliates are the AABB, the Red Cross, the Council of Community Blood Centers, the American Hospital Association, the American Medical Association, and the Blue Cross Association. The donor and consumer representatives include the American Heart Association, the AFL-CIO, the American Legion, the National Kidney Association, the United Auto Workers, and the United Way of America. Table 9.1 lists the current members.

Despite the impressive membership list, the American Blood Commission has not accomplished its prime task. The Red Cross and the AABB still stand apart. Neither the participation of interested professional and voluntary groups in the Commission nor cajoling by federal officials has overcome all the serious differences between the two major collection organizations.

The American Blood Commission is not, however, without important achievements. It furthered the development and field testing of a uniform blood-labeling system that should reduce transfusion errors and, when fully adopted, permit better tracking of blood units. A National Blood Data Center has been created as an affiliate of the Commission to collect information on blood banking and blood utilization. It has begun providing the blood-banking community with the types of comprehensive and comparative statistics common in the health field but never available in blood banking.

Considerable progress has been made in the development of coordinated regional blood programs. The very discussion of criteria for an organization to be recognized by the ABC as a regional provider of blood services has forced many blood centers, includ-

Table 9.1 Membership of American Blood Commission 1981–1982.

Professional organizations	Donor and consumer organizations
Am. Assoc. of Blood Banks	Am. Assoc. Donor Recruitment Professionals
Am. Assoc. Clin. Histocompat. Testing	Am. Cancer Society
Am. Assoc. Tissue Banks	AFL-CIO
Am. Coll. Emerg. Physicians	Am. Heart Assoc.
Am. Coll. of Physicians	Am. Legion
Am. Coll. of Surgeons	Communications Workers of America
Am. Hospital Assoc.	Cooley's Anemia Found.
Am. Medical Assoc.	Leukemia Soc. of America
Am. Nurses' Assoc.	Nat. Assoc. of Patients on Hemodialysis and Transplant.
Am. Osteopathic Assoc.	Nat. Assoc. of Sickle Cell Disease
Am. Osteopathic Coll.	
Am. Red Cross	Nat. Hemophilia Found.
Am. Soc. Anesthesiologists	Nat. Kidney Found.
Am. Soc. Clin. Path.	Nat. Retired Teachers Assoc.– Am. Assoc. Retired Persons
Am. Soc. Hematol.	
Am. Surgical Assoc.	United Auto Workers
Blue Cross Assoc.	United Way of America
Coll. of Am. Path.	
Council of Comm. Blood Centers	
Health Insur. Assoc. of America	
Nat. Medical Assoc.	
Pharm. Manufacturers Assoc.	
Soc. of Cryobiology	
Veterans Administration	

ing no small number of Red Cross blood centers, to become much more responsible suppliers.

However, the American Blood Commission has many problems, not the least of which is money. Despite its origin—a not too immaculate conception achieved under strong governmental pressure—the ABC is legally a private-sector organization that must, to meet some of its financial needs, compete for grants and contracts from the government. No governmental agency either has or seeks responsibility for ensuring the financial viability of the ABC. No public appropriation is earmarked for it. Instead, the ABC must rely mainly on the willingness of its members to donate funds for its maintenance. Yet to most of its members blood banking is a peripheral issue—perhaps a civic obligation, but not a central concern. Only the blood-collection organizations and a few specialized client groups have blood banking high enough on their organizational agendas to merit priority in their budgetary obligations. Blood-collection organizations, however, can also see the ABC as a battleground and threaten to withhold payments in their continuing interorganizational conflict. Not surprisingly, as nearly half of the ABC's budget is provided by the major blood-banking organizations, it lives in perpetual uncertainty over its financial viability.

Few opportunities to express interorganizational hostility are missed. In 1976 the Red Cross announced its intention to terminate its participation in the blood clearinghouse system, in which it had been active since 1960. The reasons cited included the shipment to commercial blood banks of blood collected by the Red Cross and other complex consequences of the manner in which the Clearinghouse settled its accounts. More fundamentally, the Red Cross was objecting to the use of blood credits of any type, a topic then under discussion within the ABC Donor Recruitment Task Force. With its bold act, the Red Cross hoped to force a realignment in blood-collection practices that would bring the practices of all collectors into conformity with its own mode of intended operation.

Eventually, the Donor Recruitment Task Force did recommend that all whole-blood collections move toward community responsibility and away from the use of such devices as nonreplacement fees and blood credits. The proposal was endorsed in a split vote by the ABC Board. The Red Cross was joined in its support of the recommendation by the Council of Community Blood Centers and by nearly all of the consumer and donor organizations represented on the board. Vigorous dissent by the AABB and several health-service organizations has limited efforts at implementation, and appeared for about a year to threaten the survival of the ABC. Given its structure, it is difficult for the ABC to undertake anything of serious consequence without the approval of both the Red Cross and the AABB. The outcomes of their cooperative and competitive efforts remain the key to blood banking in the United States.

That the Red Cross and the AABB continue to sit together and often to work together is seen by some as a promising sign. There are issues on which they are in general agreement. Both the Red Cross and the AABB favor eliminating the practice of paying for blood donations and, not incidentally, the competition from commercial collectors. Like the Red Cross, the larger blood centers that dominate the AABB also can see advantages in regionalization. Already several banks have claimed the status of and been designated by the ABC as regional banks, responsible for the coordination of collections and the provision of a full spectrum of specialized blood services within a defined territory.

These common interests, rather than the threat of direct governmental intervention, have kept the ABC functioning. The major blood-banking organizations know too much about Washington politics to believe that punitive legislation is likely to be used to restructure a blood-collection system that is managed by nonprofit agencies and that lacks a genuine crisis. They are certainly aware that the mandate governmental officials possess to promote the national blood policy was the result of the passing initiative of one Secretary of Health, Education, and Welfare and has not been renewed by his several successors. But each finds the threat convenient for its own purposes—the Red Cross blood program to gain independence from other Red Cross activities, the AABB to discipline its many small institutional members, and the CCBC to share equal standing with its larger rivals. They all look forward to a more regionalized blood-banking system.

To maintain organizational harmony, the ABC has not pressed regional units to conform to all its policies, especially the one concerned with the elimination of the nonreplacement fee. Although this may disturb some advocates of reform, the Red Cross has been able to accommodate it for the time being. The ABC has had promising working groups on "Resource Sharing" (arrangements for interregional movement of blood resources as an alternative to the original AABB Clearinghouse system). The idea of regionalization, the recognition of local dominance, has great appeal within the Red Cross, as it does among the larger AABB and CCBC units. Whether regionalization will prove to be a desirable trend in blood banking is an issue to which we shall return.

Controlling Hepatitis

Whatever the outcome of the conflict between the Red Cross and its opponents, organizational changes are not likely to offer a solution to the hepatitis problem. Some technical progress, however, is being made. A third-generation screening test based on the hepatitis B surface antigen has already been widely disseminated and can be credited with some of the decline that is noted in transfusion-related disease. A hepatitis vaccine is under development, promising eventual protection from the disease for certain groups (such as medical personnel and homosexuals) particularly at risk of contracting it. Unfortunately, the prospects for effectively using the vaccine in preventing post-transfusion hepatitis by immunizing donors or patients are dubious.

The non-A, non-B type of hepatitis, apparently the most prevalent form of the disease transmitted by blood transfusions, is not yet well understood. In the United States and abroad intensive research is being conducted to identify the agents responsible for the generation of this type of hepatitis. Although incremental progress in this effort has been reported, most researchers would agree that the development of appropriate screening tests and vaccines is not yet on the horizon.

Other technical approaches to the reduction of the hepatitis problem are also being pursued. Frozen-red-cell technology, originally introduced to extend greatly the useful storage lifetime of red cells in order to facilitate the management of transfusion facilities, is now thought by some to offer advantages over whole blood with respect to hepatitis. Studies indicate that the freezing of red cells does not in itself eliminate the risk of hepatitis transmission; rather it appears that the thawing process, which involves washing away preservatives, results in a product that is somewhat less risky than whole blood. Careful calibration of such effects, however, would require extensive prospective studies, which may or may not be worth the cost given the present level of the hepatitis problem.

Also under investigation are substances that are being referred to as "artificial blood." When infused into the body's circulatory system, these substances can bind oxygen and therefore can serve as oxygen-transfer agents in the manner of whole blood. As synthetic compounds they would carry no risk of hepatitis. In conjunction with albumin, a safe blood-volume expander obtained from plasma donations, the availability of an artificial oxygen-transfer agent would offer a hepatitis-free set of compounds that could provide the major therapeutic functions sought in most blood transfusions. Initial tests of artificial blood in animals, however, have been only marginally successful, indicating that more development is needed.

Taken together, the technical attacks on hepatitis are impressive. Although no sure means of prevention are at hand, several promising avenues are being explored. We are convinced that it will be one or another of these developments rather than any further effort at social reform that will make transfusions safe from hepatitis-induced illness and death.

The Pharmaceutical Sector

A market for whole-blood donation no longer exists in the United States. Its elimination brought about some improvement in hepatitis rates, but did not produce peace among the major blood collectors. The removal of money exchanges for whole-blood donations does appear to have satisfied those who are outraged by the use of money as an incentive for the gift of life. But money is still exchanged in the collection of blood plasma, also vital for life. Will plasma collections provide the next major public blood-banking controversy?

As we noted, the structure of plasma collections differs sharply from that of whole-blood collections, both in this country and in most others that collect plasma by pheresis. Most plasma donors are paid, and the bulk of the collections are made by private profit-making collectors that are either subsidiaries of or suppliers to major drug firms that process plasma into blood pharmaceuticals. Voluntary plasmapheresis donations are few, partially because the gift is a much less convenient one and partially because the nonprofit whole-blood collectors have shown little enthusiasm for taking responsibility for the plasma supply. Volunteer plasma is of course obtained from whole blood donations, but much of it is used for direct transfusion and far too little is left to meet the needs for source material for blood pharmaceuticals. Primarily a commercial activity, and relying upon repeat paid donors, plasma collections are not very visible to the general public. Rare are the posters seeking plasma donors.

This system seems to work extraordinarily well in providing an acceptable supply of plasma. Indeed, the United States collects sufficient plasma internally to meet not only its own medical needs, but also part of the needs of the rest of the world. Many countries have banned commercial plasma collections and then proved unable to meet their needs through voluntary, unpaid plasma donations. Several major plasma collectors and processors in the United States are now owned by foreign firms, which may indicate the strategy to which some nations resort to meet their needs for plasma-based pharmaceuticals.

Most plasma derivatives do not transmit disease. The major exceptions are those derivatives useful in treating hemophilia, derivatives for which there is no safe substitute. (Hemophiliacs appear, however, to develop greater resistance to hepatitis transmission than most other classes of blood-product recipients.) As opposed to the situation that held for some commercial whole-blood collectors, there is no clear evidence that commercial plasma collectors bring unnecessary risk to the patients who receive their products. There is, however, the fear that plasmapheresis donations, induced by an immediate financial reward, can result in some donors knowingly or unknowingly placing themselves in jeopardy by donating either too often or in the presence of other limitations on their health. Some plasmapheresis donor populations seem too easily exploited. However, collectors are now required to be licensed by the Food and Drug Administration, the agency whose responsibilities include setting standards for and monitoring the health effects of plasma donations. So far, donations made within FDA guidelines appear to be safe. Any other plasmapheresis donations would be illegal.

Plasma apparently is not a very profitable business. As basic pharmaceuticals, the plasma products produced by the different manufacturers must be functionally identical. Thus, cutting manufacturing costs becomes the key to market success. The recent leveling off of the demand for many plasma products has brought excess production capacity and price reductions. Competition for market share among the plasma processors is intense. It is, however, a quiet undertaking. Without significant participation by nonprofit organizations, there is not the conflict over jurisdiction and philosophy found in whole-blood collections.

This quiet may not last. New "fast membrane" technologies for plasmapheresis are developing rapidly. These promise major reductions in the time required for a plasma donation, although there is likely also to be a significant increase in the cost of the disposables required for such donations. Even so, the possibility of making plasmapheresis donation much more similar to whole-blood donation makes one wonder whether issues similar to those that essentially wiped out commercial whole-blood collection will arise in the plasma sector. The shortened donation time may encourage voluntary donors to contribute plasma on a much increased scale. Thus far, however, the nonprofit whole-blood collection organizations have shown only limited interest in the processing of plasma and even less interest in testing the willingness of the American public to provide the larger part of plasma needs by voluntary donations.

Public Participation in the Whole-Blood Supply

The whole-blood supply in the United States appears to us to be in excellent condition. A large part of the adult population responds generously to well-organized collection programs that combine convenient donation opportunities with reasonably personal forms of donor solicitation. We estimate that about half the people who are now eligible to donate blood have done so at least once. The continuing need for an adequate blood supply is well understood, both because of the solicitation information provided in the media and because most adults are aware of at least one personal acquaintance who has been the recipient of a blood transfusion.

Provision of an adequate whole-blood supply requires, on the average, about one donation every seven years from every eligible potential blood donor. Because many active donors give their blood more than once a year, about 3.5 percent of the population of the United States, or about 10 percent of those eligible to donate, make whole-blood donations during any particular year. The limited number of blood donors during any year is more a consequence of the level of medical needs for blood than of public willingness to participate voluntarily in the whole-blood supply.

With the exception of a few special cases, such as New York City (still heavily dependent on the importation of red cells from Europe) and Miami (where a major blood center went into receivership), most regions of this country have a dependable whole-blood supply obtained largely from donors within the regions. It seems unlikely that more than about 3 percent of the whole-blood supply is obtained by monetary payment; some of this paid-for blood is obtained by elite medical institutions to meet special needs.

The growth rate of blood needs, although irregular, is mild relative to the number of experienced and willing donors. Furthermore, most nondonors who are medically eligible to give believe they have not made firm decisions to remain nondonors. Medical needs for blood are far below any level that might exceed the willingness of the public to provide whole blood. And yet, the blood system is not invulnerable. To function properly it requires dedicated people and efficient organizations. More important, it requires the public's trust, which must be earned and sustained.

The Integrity of Public Information

The Achilles' heel of the whole-blood supply as it now operates in the United States is the integrity of the messages conveyed to the public about blood. Journalists and the media display what they judge to be good citizenship in supporting a public function as important as the provision of the whole-blood supply. One consequence of these good intentions is that whatever messages blood centers wish to distribute are passed along as "news" to the public with less documentation and fewer questions than may be appropriate. Although the problem has diminished in most parts of the country, the too-frequent "blood shortage emergencies" are one potential type of abuse of the public-information channels available to blood centers. Acts of nature and catastrophic accidents can give rise to extreme blood needs and emergency appeals even in the best managed collection and distribution systems. In some regions, however, there has been a tendency to substitute dramatic media appeals in place of adequate planning for blood supplies during the holiday and vacation periods. A few recent examples of the critical review of such appeals by the press remind us of the frail nature of recruitment systems that "cry wolf" too often.

As some regional blood programs achieve the competence to collect more whole blood than their regions require, public service and financial considerations encourage the export of surplus blood to other regions with less adequate collection systems. In the short run, this practice benefits both the exporting and the importing regional blood programs. Nevertheless, it seems that, if a region consistently exports blood, the local population deserves to be informed of the level of export of their freely donated blood and of future export plans. If interregional "resource sharing" is to prevail in a manner requiring an average outflow from certain regions, the local population may wish to set some upper bound on how much of their blood may be collected for export. At the very least, we believe that sustained resource sharing on a national level requires both informed donor consent and some assurance that regions that are consistent importers are doing everything possible to develop their indigenous whole-blood supplies. Age distributions and geographical properties of some regions may always limit their internal blood collections, but we think it important that places such as Miami and New York City develop indigenous blood supplies if populations elsewhere are to be willing to provide their blood for the temporary assistance of such regions. We agree that, in the end, blood is a national (or international) resource. Yet we expect that there are and should be limits on the degree to which donors in one region are willing to subsidize the blood needs of other regions that take inadequate responsibility for developing their own blood collections.

There are other aspects of the integrity of blood-related information. The public is often misinformed, as often by accident as by intent, about the "benefits" offered to blood donors in return for their blood. Because of the length and complexity of the donor solicitation chain, for example, many community-responsibility collection systems are still misinforming their donors with allegations of various forms of "blood insurance" benefits. Similarly, some individual-responsibility systems at least imply that blood availability is likely to be affected by an individual or a group's past contributions to the blood supply. These misleading messages still exist. Although the donors may not care much one way or the other, the long-term credibility of the whole blood-collection system must eventually be compromised by lying to an intelligent and supportive public.

Collection Ideology

In a well-administered blood-collection environment, people's decisions about donation seem to be relatively simple, driven above all by recognition of the continuing medical need for an adequate supply of human blood. We have no reason to believe that individual- and community-responsibility blood systems attract different types of donors.

Although ideological differences have served as public focal points for disputes between the major blood-collection organizations, it is clear from experience that a reasonably coordinated regional blood program can meet blood needs comfortably under either individual-responsibility or community-responsibility arrangements. Although changes from one system to the other can be difficult to explain and implement, the underlying ideological issues are not of much concern to the public. Even many ardent blood donors are neither well-informed nor concerned about the ideological basis under which their blood is collected and distributed.

The nonreplacement fee may once have been a helpful device for small hospitals attempting to collect their own whole-blood supplies, but today the fee is far more a fiscal than a recruitment tool, with little effect on a region's ability to meet its blood needs. By design, individual-responsibility systems lead to a less uniform distribution of charges to patients who require blood transfusions. Many blood-collection messages and practices are surprisingly similar in both types of systems.

At a slow but observable rate, an irreversible movement toward regional blood-collection systems based entirely on community responsibility, as recommended by the American Blood Commission, appears well underway. Whether this regionalization benefits the public will depend upon the seriousness with which the managers of the system take their responsibility. The fact that the blood-supply system is approaching the reliability and integration of the water-supply system is encouraging; but given the problems that can befall even a public utility as simple in purpose and structure as the water supply, no one should wish that the performance of blood banking ever be taken for granted.

Cartelization and its Consequences

A common ground among the major blood-collection centers is their interest in regional domination. The efforts of the American Blood Commission to encourage regionalization serve the interests of the larger blood centers, both within and outside the Red Cross. A secure jurisdiction is, after all, the quest of every organization.

The history of blood banking in the United States is a history of interorganizational conflict. The Red Cross sought, but failed to achieve, a national monopoly in whole-blood collections. Efforts to reconcile the Red Cross with its rivals were unsuccessful, as each held hope that it would gain dominance over the others. A similar and often intense competition for control appeared in many locales.

Paralleling the interorganizational conflict, there has been no shortage of intraorganizational conflict. Within the Red Cross a struggle has existed between the blood program and the organization's many other activities and needs. In particular, the highly professional needs of blood banking have been difficult to accommodate within the voluntary structure of the Red Cross. The AABB has its own difficulties, including tension between its larger blood centers and the blood banks at many individual hospitals. One example of this tension was the formation of the Council of Community Blood Centers by a group of centers that found the AABB unable to represent some of their primary concerns.

Many of these conflicts have been alleviated. In most metropolitan areas a single blood center has achieved something close to total dominance of the whole-blood supply. In other areas there has been an amalgamation of, or at least more coordination among, rival units. The Red Cross has given its blood program some of the independence it seeks. A great many hospitals have abandoned their efforts to fill some or all of their own blood needs. Nationally, a generation of blood bankers is passing, and with it will go a great deal of the antagonism between the Red Cross and the AABB. In place of the antagonism, there is a growing professionalism within blood banking—a professionalism that sees advantage in cooperation and coordination.

No doubt the decline of conflict will encourage more regionalization as each large blood bank seeks national recognition of its local dominance. This policy is in line with the desires of federal officials and those of the ABC, which acts as the certifier of regional status.

But there are dangers in regionalization despite its contribution to interorganizational harmony. Blood collection and the provision of routine blood services are repetitious, dull, and often exhausting tasks. Each regional center is by definition a supplier of specialized blood and tissue services. Large centers are likely to have directors who are senior physicians with intense research interests. It is the research and the specialized services rather than the blood collections that attract research support, organizational prestige, and public interest.

Determining the allocation of resources between routine services and more exotic activities is a complex issue. By intent or accident, the director of a major blood center is likely to overpower his board of directors by virtue of his knowledge and prominence and the inability of the directors to make firsthand comparisons with practices at other blood centers. Even the priorities of medical advisory boards, unless the membership is carefully controlled, are likely to emphasize research and medical progress over more conventional service. The danger is that regional blood centers may grow neglectful of their obligation to provide adequate routine blood supplies efficiently.

Although this danger is not new, it rises in importance as the regional centers gain monopoly status. Hospital blood banks have less bargaining power after they relinquish their own blood-collection activities. Most members of the public no longer have any choice among blood collectors. If regional centers do not show adequate integrity and appreciation in dealing with their local populations, donors unhappy with the regional center are likely to become ex-donors; they have no alternative blood collectors. Vigilance is required to prevent large blood programs from becoming impersonal monoliths. Much of this vigilance has been provided recently. Some major blood programs are meeting the challenge of organizing and sustaining dependable donor bases to meet local needs. But that attention to the blood-giving public must be maintained after the challenging task has been accomplished, and that will prove harder to do. The cartelization of blood banking in the United States, which regionalization implies, necessitates the creation of effective public oversight mechanisms.

The antitrust laws protect the public from the consequences of collusion among profit-making organizations. They embody the belief that the consumer suffers when competition fades. No such protection exists in the conduct of charitable, nonprofit activities. If blood banking is to be removed from the rigors of rivalry and the pressures of commercial competition, then we must worry about its performance.

As we have seen in the case of the American Blood Commission, self-regulation is inadequate. The larger collectors hold *de facto* veto power over the activities of the organization. The success of the private sector's efforts to achieve regionalization, ironically, will lead to more public regulation of blood banking, not less. Once blood banking is totally cartelized, the public interest will require governmental monitoring of the performance of the industry, just as in every other case of a private monopoly of a vital public service.

Notes

Chapter 1

1. The $2 billion annual cost figure for the products and services provided by the blood-services complex in the United States is a conservative lower bound obtained by simple estimates of the total amount charged to hospital patients for transfusions and blood products and the dollar value of the products of the blood-pharmaceutical industry.

2. Hearing before the Subcommittee on Health and Scientific Research of the Committee on Labor and Human Resources, U.S. Senate, first session to assess the progress of the National Blood Policy, June 7, 1979 document 49-656 0 (Washington, D.C.: U.S. Government Printing Office).

3. Richard M. Titmuss, *The Gift Relationship* (London: Allen and Unwin, 1969; New York: Pantheon, 1971). The publication of this book was followed by a deluge of commentary about blood collection ideology. Some examples are Kenneth J. Arrow, "Gifts and Exchanges," *Philos. and Public Affairs* 1: 343–362 (1972); Nathan Glazer, "Blood," *Public Interest* 24: 86–94 (1971); Phillip Morrison, book review, *Sci. Am.*, June 1971: 131; Paul A. Samuelson, "Blood—British and American Policies," *Newsweek* 78: 94 (1971); and Robert M. Solow, "Blood and Thunder," *Yale Law Rev.* 80: 1696–1711 (1971). The stream of commentary and letters to journals continued for several years.

4. Robert Massie and Suzanne Massie, *Journey* (New York: Knopf, 1975).

5. Sources of present and past blood-donation statistics are discussed in chapter 7.

6. National Blood Data Center, 1979 Annual Census (Washington, D.C.: National Blood Data Center, 1980).

7. American Blood Commission, Annual Report, 1979–1980 and Five Year Review 1975–1980 (Washington, D.C.: American Blood Commission, 1980).

8. There are no sound bases for a convincing estimate of paid whole-blood collections prior to 1971. Although more recent data may provide leads to the fraction of the whole-blood supply obtained from "commercial collectors," the purchase of blood by hospitals and other noncommercial collectors is often not accounted for. A major study in 1971, for example, estimated that about 11 percent of whole-blood collections were obtained by commercial collectors. With many hospitals and at least several blood centers paying some of their donors, it seems likely that more than 20 percent of the whole blood collected was obtained from paid donors in 1971. See Summary Report, NHLI's Blood Resource Studies, DHEW publication (NIH) 73-416 (Bethesda, Md.: U.S. Department of Health, Education, and Welfare, 1972). No major blood centers

and very few hospitals pay any whole-blood donors at the present time. Most commercial whole-blood collectors either closed or went into other fields (such as plasmapheresis) in the 1970s. See also chapter 6.

9. Reference 7, p. 6.

10. Bruce A. Friedman, Trudy L. Burns, and M. Anthony Schork, A Study of National Trends in Transfusion Practice (Ann Arbor, Mich.: University of Michigan Medical School and School of Public Health, 1980).

11. K. S. Abramowitz and L. A. Sanders, Baxter Travenol Laboratories —Analysis of Blood Collection Equipment Industry and Implications for the Fenwal Division (New York: Sanford C. Bernstein and Company, 1978.)

Chapter 2

1. They can also debate whether individual responsibility incentives are more likely to lead blood donors to misrepresent their health status, compromising either their own health or the safety of the blood supply. We know of no evidence of either problem resulting from conventional IR practices. The health consequences of monetary payment to blood donors is reviewed in chapter 4.

2. Both the Red Cross and the American Blood Commission have taken strong positions (discussed in chapter 9) in support of community-responsibility practices. Their recommendations have been implemented slowly but steadily. Whether the resulting practices are to be CR-SG or IR-SG depends primarily on the degree of solicitation applied to visitors and other associates of hospital patients.

3. Written solicitation material prepared for individual collection sites, usually by well-meaning volunteers, normally has an overwhelming dose of individual-responsibility messages. Examples appear all the time, even for industrial and school drives within CR-SG regions. Friends around the country who are aware of the authors' interests often mail us frighteningly powerful IR solicitation materials from blood drives within CR-SG programs.

Chapter 3

1. There are no strong bases for estimating annual whole-blood collections before the late 1960s. A helpful review of what is known appears in Paul D. Cumming, National Blood Policy and the American Blood Commission: A Systems Study, Ph.D. diss., State University of New York at Buffalo, 1976. Estimates of more recent annual blood collections are discussed in chapter 7.

2. For an interesting social history of the evolution of blood banking in the United States, concerned in part with how the ideologies of regional blood practices were determined, see Louanne Kennedy, Community

Blood Banking in the United States 1937–1975: Organization, Formation, Transformation, and Reform in a Climate of Competition, Ph.D. diss., New York University, 1978.

3. Although there are still many institutions collecting whole blood in the Houston area, considerable progress has been made in establishing a regional center and in coordinating collections during the last five or so years. Chicago has several major blood collectors but, we believe, less coordination. Attempts at a Chicago Regional Blood Program have not made much progress. There are few major metropolitan areas in which the great majority of blood services are not provided by a single blood center and its regional blood program.

4. A nontechnical discussion of present collection planning and inventory-management practice is Douglas M. Surgenor, "Managing The Dynamics of the Blood Supply System," in Words at Detroit, Blood Services Management Conference (Washington, D.C.: American National Red Cross, 1980), pp. 3–18.

5. More recently, it is the case that only 8 out of the 57 Red Cross regional blood programs provide less than 90 percent of their regions' blood needs. The majority provide total blood supply for their hospitals.

6. The Puget Sound Blood Center in the state of Washington has at times stored all its inventory in its own blood banks, delivering blood to hospitals only after crossmatches are accomplished. Major hospitals have functioned well without any blood inventory. This arrangement and the logistics required to maintain it are extremely uncommon.

7. Attempts by the American Blood Commission to gain federal support for a major study of the effectiveness of blood-supply utilization failed. See Freedman, Burns, and Schork (chapter 1, ref. 10) for a unique report on hospital blood-use statistics.

Chapter 4

1. Between 1966 and 1976 the average number of reported cases of hepatitis was slightly over 55,000 according to *Morbidity and Mortality Wkly. Rep.* 26, no. 22: 177 (1977).

2. Center for Disease Control, Hepatitis Surveillance Report 36, U.S. Department of Health, Education, and Welfare, Public Health Service, 1973, pp. 20–21.

3. Alfred M. Prince, Betsy Brofman, George F. Grady, William J. Kuhns, Charles Zazzi, Richard W. Levine, and Stephen J. Millian, "Posttransfusion Viral Hepatitis Caused by an Agent or Agents Other than Hepatitis B virus or Hepatitis A virus. Impact on Efficiency of Present Screening Methods," in Tibor J. Greenwalt and Graham A. Jamieson (eds.), *Transmissible Disease and Blood Transfusion* (New York: Grune and Stratton, 1975), pp. 129–140; James W. Mosley, Allan G. Redeker, S. M. Feinstone, and R. M. Purcell, "Multiple Hepatitis Viruses in Multiple Attacks of

Acute Viral Hepatitis," *N. Engl. J. Med.* 296: 75–78 (1977); Saul Krugman, "Viral Hepatitis: Recent Developments and Prospects for Prevention," *J. Pediatrics* 87: 1067 (1975).

4. John A. Bryan and Michael B. Gregg, "Viral Hepatitis in the United States (1970–1973): An Analysis of Morbidity Trends and the Impact of HBsAg Testing on Surveillance and Epidemiology," *Am. J. Med. Sci.* 270: 271 (1975); H. J. Alter, P. V. Holland, and R. H. Purcell, "The Emerging Pattern of Post-Transfusion Hepatitis," *Am. J. Med. Sci.* 279: 329 (1975).

5. B. S. Blumberg, H. J. Allen, and S. Visnich, "A 'New' Antigen in Leukemia Sera," *JAMA* 191: 541 (1965).

6. G. L. Giorgioni, F. B. Hollinger, L. LeDuc, S. Issarescu, J. George, A. Blackman, and W. R. Thayer, "Radioimmunoassay Detection of Hepatitis Type B Antigen," *JAMA* 222: 1514 (1972).

7. R. H. Russell and J. L. Gerin, "Hepatitis B Subunit Vaccine: A Preliminary Report of Safety and Efficacy Tests in Chimpanzees," *Am. J. Med. Sci.* 270: 395 (1975).

8. M. Goldfield, H. C. Black, J. Bill, S. Sringhongse, and W. Pizzuti, "The Consequences of Administering Blood Pretested for HBsAg by Third Generation Techniques: A Progress Report," *Am. J. Med. Sci.* 270: 335 (1975).

9. S. M. Feinstone, A. Z. Kapilian, R. H. Purcell, H. J. Alter, and P. V. Holland, "Transfusion-Associated Hepatitis Not Due to Viral Hepatitis Type A or B," *N. Engl. J. Med.* 292: 767 (1975); Prince et al., ref. 3.

10. Richard D. Aach, Wolf Szmuness, James W. Mosley, F. Blaine Hollinger, Richard A. Kahn, Cladd E. Stevens, Virginia M. Edwards, and Jochewed Werch, "Serum Alanine Aminotransferase of Donors in Relation to the Risk of Non-A, Non-B Hepatitis in Recipients: The Transfusion-Transmitted Viruses Study," *N. Engl. J. Med.* 304:989–994 (1981).

11. Attributed to CDC or DHEW Assistant Secretary for Health estimates in *Hepatitis from Blood Transfusions: Evaluation of Methods to Reduce the Problem*, Report to the Congress by the Comptroller General of the United States, MND-75-82, 1976, pp. 2–3.

12. For example, see H. F. Taswell, R. Shorter, T. K. Poncelet, and N. G. Maxwell, "Hepatitis-Associated Antigen in Blood Donor Population," *JAMA* 214: 142 (1980); L. B. Seeff, E. C. Wright, H. J. Zimmerman, and R. W. McCallum, *Am. J. Med. Sci.* 270: 335 (1975).

13. R. S. Koff, T. C. Chalmers, P. O. Culhane, F. L. Iber, and the Boston Inter-Hospital Liver Group, "Underreporting of Viral Hepatitis," *Gastroenterology* 64: 1194 (1973).

14. Office of the Assistant Secretary for Health, Department of Health, Education, and Welfare, Posttransfusion Hepatitis—Cases, Deaths, and Costs, unpublished paper, 1973.

15. G. F. Grady, A. J. E. Bennett, and the National Transfusion Hepatitis Study, "Risk of Posttransfusion Hepatitis in the United States," *JAMA* 220: 692–702 (1972).

16. M. J. Goldfield, An Epidemiologic Study of Transfusion-Associated Hepatitis, unpublished report, New Jersey State Department of Health, 1976.

17. Dependence of Massachusetts Blood Banks on Paid Donors, 1971, unpublished paper, Massachusetts Department of Public Health, Division of Medical Care, 1972; P. W. Holley and B. Y. Linkenhofer, *JAMA* 234: 1051 (1975); ref. 11 above.

18. For example, see H. J. Alter, R. H. Purcell, S. M. Feinstone, P. V. Holland, and A. G. Morrow, "Non-A/Non-B Hepatitis: A Review and Interim Report of an Ongoing Prospective Study," in G. N. Vyas, S. N. Cohen, and R. Schmid (eds.), *Viral Hepatitis* (Philadelphia: Franklin Institute Press, 1978).

19. C. M. Kunin, "Serum Hepatitis from Whole Blood: Incidence and Relation to Source of Blood," *Am. J. Med. Sci.* 237: 293 (1959).

20. J. Garrot Allen, *The Epidemiology of Posttransfusion Hepatitis: Basic Blood and Plasma Tabulations*, 1972; J. Garrot Allen, "Commercially Obtained Blood and Serum Hepatitis," *Surgery, Gynecology, and Obstetrics* 131: 277 (1970).

21. H. J. Alter, P. V. Holland, R. H. Purcell, J. J. Lander, S. M. Feinstone, A. G. Morrow, and P. I. Schmidt, "Posttransfusion Hepatitis After Inclusions of Commercial and Hepatitis-B Antigen-Positive Donors," *Ann. Internal Med.* 77: 691–699 (1972).

22. M. J. Goldfield, An Epidemiologic Study of Transfusion-Associated Hepatitis, progress reports for November 1975–December 1976 and July 1973–February 1974, New Jersey Department of Health.

23. J. B. Alsever and P. B. Van Schoonhoven, "Posttransfusion Viral Hepatitis (PTVH): Myths and Facts," *Arizona Med.* 31: 253 (1974).

24. W. Szmuness, R. L. Hirsch, A. M. Prince, R. W. Levine, E. J. Harley, and H. Ikram, "Hepatitis B Surface Antigen in Blood Donors: Further Observations," *J. Infectious Diseases* 131: 111–118 (1975).

25. Summary statement of Ad Hoc Committee on Alanine Amino Transferase Testing of Blood Donors, coordinated by the National Heart, Lung, and Blood Institute, July 1981.

26. "Screening of Blood Donors for Non-A Non-B Hepatitis" (editorial), *Lancet*, July 11, 1981.

27. L. R. Bryant, "Use of Frozen-Thawed Deglycerolized Red Blood Cells in Community Clinical Practice," in R. B. Dawson and A. Barnes, Jr. (eds.), *Clinical and Practical Aspects of the Use of Frozen Blood: A Technical Workshop* (Atlanta: American Association of Blood Banks, 1977), pp. 77–97; S. Sumida, "Frozen Blood and Hepatitis," *Cryobiology* 13: 657–658 (1976); M. Telischi, R. Hoiberg, and K. R. P. Rao, "The Use of Frozen, Thawed Erythrocytes in Blood Banking," *Am. J. Clin. Pathol.* 68: 250–257 (1977); M. J. Wooten, "Use and Analysis of Saline Washed Red Blood Cells," *Transfusion* 16: 464–468 (1976).

28. R. K. Haugen, "Hepatitis After the Transfusion of Frozen Red Cells and Washed Red Cells," *N. Engl. J. Med.* 301: 393–395 (1979); H. J. Alter, E. Tabor, H. T. Meryman, J. H. Hoofnagle, R. A. Kahn, P. V. Holland, R. J. Gerety, and L. F. Barker, "Transmission of Hepatitis-B Virus Infection by Transfusion of Frozen Deglycerolized Red Blood Cells," *N. Engl. J. Med.* 298: 637–642 (1978).

29. J. H. Hoofnagle and L. F. Barker, "Hepatitis B Virus and Albumin Products," in Proceedings of the Workshop on Albumin, DHEW publication (NIH) 76-925 (1976). Guidelines for protective practices for blood collection and transfusion appear as "Blood Services Directives" of the American Red Cross and in the "Standards for Blood Banks and Transfusion Services" of the American Association of Blood Banks. Both of these are revised and reissued frequently. Protective regulations as promulgated by the Bureau of Biologics of the Food and Drug Administration appear in 21 Code of Federal Regulations, parts 600–799, and are published in the *Federal Register* when changes are made.

30. P. J. Schmidt, "Transfusion Mortality; with Special Reference to Surgical and Intensive Care Facilities," *J. Florida Med. Assn.* 67: 151–153 (1980).

31. B. Myrhe, *Quality Control in Blood Banking* (New York: Wiley, 1974).

32. Bruce A. Friedman, Trudy L. Burns and M. Anthony Schork, A Study of National Trends in Transfusion Practice (Ann Arbor: University of Michigan School of Medicine and School of Public Health, 1980).

Chapter 5

1. Brigadier General Douglas B. Kendrick, Blood Program in World War II (Washington, D.C.: Medical Department, United States Army, 1964), pp. 101–137. The American Red Cross and other organizations had been collecting plasma for British needs since 1940.

2. 33 Stat. 599, as amended; 36 U.S.C. 1. Note also "The American National Red Cross," *The United States Government Manual 1978/79* (Washington, D.C.: Office of the Federal Register, 1979), pp. 849–852.

3. Foster R. Dulles, *The American Red Cross* (New York: Harper & Row, 1950; Westport, Conn.: Greenwood, 1971).

4. The effect of governmentally provided welfare on private charity is worldwide. See Lord Allen of Abbeydale, "Some Problems Facing Charities," *Three Banks Rev.* no. 114 (June 1977): 28–41 for an analysis of the British situation since the rise of the welfare state.

5. Dulles, *American Red Cross*, p. 527.

6. Dulles, *American Red Cross*, p. 529, apparently quoting an internal Red Cross memorandum.

7. "Historical Highlights of ARC Participation in Blood Programs," in Staff Study Report, National Blood Program (Washington, D.C.: Ameri-

can National Red Cross, January, 1952), chap. 1, pp. 42–43. Note also G. F. McGinnes, "National Blood Program of the American Red Cross," *Am. J. Public Health* 39: 1429–1430 (1949).

8. Staff Study National Blood Program (ref. 7), pp. 39–40.

9. Staff Study National Blood Program (ref. 7), p. 43.

10. Dulles, *American Red Cross*, p. 529.

11. Staff Study National Blood Program (ref. 7), p. 43.

12. Staff Study National Blood Program (ref. 7), chap. 2, p. iii.

13. Board of Governors of the American National Red Cross, January 19, 1952, meeting transcript.

14. Board of Governors of the American National Red Cross, June 22, 1952, meeting transcript (includes a discussion of the financial arrangements involved in the support of the blood program).

15. Comments of Mr. O'Connor, Board of Governors of the American National Red Cross, December 6, 1948, meeting transcript.

16. Louanne Kennedy, Community Blood Banking in the United States From 1937–1975: Organization, Formation, Transformation, and Reform in a Climate of Competition, Ph.D. diss., New York University, 1978.

17. "Red Cross Answers its Critics," *Look*, March 28, 1961, pp. 83–87; R. Carter, "The Controversial Red Cross," *Holiday*, February 1960, pp. 80 ff.

18. Proceedings of Blood Bank Institute sponsored by Wm. Buchanan Blood Center of Baylor Hospital, Baker Hotel, Dallas, Texas, November 1947.

19. Kennedy (ref. 16, p. 88) describes the AABB's scientific efforts as a preemptive strategy in their interorganizational relations with the Red Cross.

20. Bernice M. Hemphill, "AABB National Clearinghouse Blood Program," *Medical Times* 98, no. 8: 101–107 (1970).

21. Kennedy, ref. 16, p. 108.

22. Dulles, *American Red Cross*, p. 529.

23. Note "Statement of Bernice M. Hemphill, President, American Association of Blood Banks," September 20, 1976, issued in response to the termination of Red Cross participation in the National Blood Clearinghouse Program.

24. Kenneth C. Fraundorf, "Competition in Blood Banking," *Public Policy* XXIII, no. 1: 219–240 (1975).

25. Staff Study National Blood Program, Appendix, p. 19, quoting Mr. Harriman.

26. Board of Governors of the American National Red Cross, April 7, 1952, meeting transcript.

27. "Blood and Blood Banking" (editorial), *JAMA* 193, no. 1 (July 5,

1965): 149–150; Ben Pearse, "What's Wrong With Our Blood Banks?" *Saturday Evening Post,* March 14, 1959, p. 96.

28. Kennedy, ref. 16, pp. 106–113.

29. Board of Governors of the American National Red Cross, February 20, 1967, meeting transcript. Interestingly, the military has called on neither the Red Cross nor the AABB for assistance since the Korean War. The entire blood needs of U.S. forces in Vietnam were met by donations from military personnel and their dependents collected by military medical personnel. One possible explanation of this self-sufficiency was to avoid a civilian mobilization effort for blood and thus calling additional public attention to the fighting. Another might have been the desire to avoid a choice between Red Cross and AABB assistance, given the conflict between the organizations. Some in the Red Cross were not unhappy with the military's decision, as it reduced Red Cross identification with the unpopular war.

30. Board of Governors of the American National Red Cross, April 23, 1967, meeting transcript.

31. National Heart and Lung Institute Blood Resources Studies, June 30, 1972, vol. 1, Federal and State Regulation of the Nation's Blood Resource, DHEW publication (NIH) 73-418; vol. 2, Supply and Use of the Nation's Blood Resource, DHEW publication (NIH) 73-419; vol. 3, A Pilot Study of Hemophilia Treatment in the United States, DHEW publication (NIH) 73-420. See also C. Holden, "Blood Banking: Money is at Root of System's Evils," *Science* 175 (24 March 1972): 1344–1348.

32. Office of the Secretary of Health, Education, and Welfare, "National Blood Policy: Proposed Implementation Plan; Request for Comments," *Federal Register* 39, no. 47, March 8, 1974: 9326–9330; address by Theodore Cooper (Acting Assistant Secretary for Health, U.S. Department of Health, Education, and Welfare) to the Inaugural Convention of the American Blood Commission, Washington, D.C., April 4, 1975.

33. Report of the Ad Hoc Group on Blood Policy Matters, American National Red Cross, February 1978, pp. 11–12, 22. Two of the 58 Red Cross Blood Centers are exceptions to the rule cited. One is managed by a regional rather than a chapter board; the other is a joint venture with the New York Blood Center, a CCBC member.

34. Report of the Ad Hoc Group on Blood Policy Matters, American National Red Cross, February 1978, pp. 24, 27, 30.

35. Report of the Ad Hoc Group on Blood Policy Matters, American National Red Cross, February 1978, p. 12.

36. "Red Cross Joins in a Blood Project," *New York Times,* March 16, 1979, p. 13; "The Red Cross: Drawing Blood From its Rivals," *Business Week,* September 11, 1978, pp. 113–114. "Red Cross Restructuring Unlimbers Blood Program for Regionalization, Sets Stage for Major Fractionation Venture With Baxter-Travenol," *Schechter Report; Blood Banks/Clinical Labs,* February 14, 1978.

Chapter 6

1. Charles A. Janeway, "Human Serum Albumin: Historical Review" and John W. Palmer, "The Evolution of Large-Scale Human Plasma Fractionation in the United States," in Proceedings of the Workshop on Albumin, DHEW publication (NIH) 76-925, 1976; Hayle B. Randolph, "Plasma, Its Derivatives and Market," *Plasma Quarterly* 1, no. 3: 74–75 (1979).

2. Douglas M. Surgenor, An Overview of Plasma Fractionation, unpublished paper, 1977.

3. Robert W. Reilly, "Highlights of the Activities of the Blood Resources Branch of NHLBI," *Plasma Quarterly* 1, no. 4: 106–107 (1979).

4. National Heart and Lung Institute, Blood Resource Studies, Summary Report, DHEW publication (NIH) 73-416, 1972, p. 77.

5. Reference 4, pp. 69–100.

6. Office of the Secretary of Health, Education, and Welfare, "National Blood Policy: Proposal Implementation Plan: Request for Comments," *Federal Register* 39, no. 47 (March 8, 1974): 9326–9330.

7. 21 Code of Federal Regulations 606. 120(b)(2), 1978.

8. Thomas C. Drees, Plasma Supply-Demand Worldwide, presented at the annual meeting of the American Association of Blood Banks, November 1980; Michael M. LeConey, "Who Needs Plasma," *Plasma Quarterly* 2, no. 3: 68–69 (1980).

9. James L. Tullis, "Albumin: Background and Use" and "Albumin: Guidelines for Clinical Use," *Plasma Quarterly* 3, no. 1: 6–7 (1981).

10. Reference 2; Jay H. Hoofnagle and Lewe Llys F. Barker, "Hepatitis B Virus and Albumin Products" and Charles P. Pattison et al., "Field Studies of Type B Hepatitis Associated with Transfusion of Plasma Protein Fraction," in Proceedings of the Workshop on Albumin, DHEW publication (NIH) 76-925, 1976.

11. Robert W. Reilly, Executive Director, American Blood Resources Association, personal communication.

12. Titmuss, *The Gift Relationship*; Mark Winiarsky, "Blood Drains Poor, Aids Rich," *National Catholic Reporter*, July 4, 1975; Washington Post, "Profiteering in Blood is Scored by WHO," May 17, 1975.

13. Jack Reasor, "Reasor on Demand," *Plasma Quarterly* 3, no. 1: 9 (1981).

14. "1981 listing of source plasma locations," *Plasma Quarterly* 3, no. 2: 53 (1981).

15. Vernon Fahle, "The Source Plasma Industry: Statistical Report, 1979," *Plasma Quarterly* 3, no. 3: 68 (1981). Another survey, reported by Robert W. Reilly in *Plasma Quarterly* 3, no. 2 (1981) corroborates the general idea; however, the numbers are slightly different.

16. Robert W. Reilly, personal communication.

17. Drees, ref. 8; Jack Reasor, "Perspective Into a Controversial Issue," *Plasma Quarterly* 1, no. 3: 82 (1979).

18. Jack M. Reasor, "Rejection and Attrition of Compensated Plasmapheresis Donors," *Plasma Quarterly* 1, no. 3: 72 (1979); Reasor, "The Compensated Plasma Donor, Further Definition," *Plasma Quarterly* 2, no. 1: 8 (1980).

19. Douglas M. Surgenor, Director, Northeast Regional Red Cross Blood Services, personal communication.

20. John E. Salvaggio, "The Effect of Prolonged Plasmapheresis in Immunoglobulins, Other Serum Proteins, Delayed Hypersensitivity and Phytohemagglutinin Induced Lymphocyte Transformation," *International Arch. Allergy and Applied Immunology* 41: 833–894 (1971); R. K. Batliwalla, "Report on 5,000 Plasmaphereses Performed on Hyperimmunized Blood Donors," *Plasma Quarterly* 2, no. 1: 13 (1980).

21. Robert W. Reilly, personal communication.

22. Robert W. Reilly, personal communication.

23. Kenneth Abramowitz, "Economics of Automation," *Plasma Quarterly* 1, no. 2: 41 (1979).

Chapter 7

1. Robert M. Oswalt, "A Review of Blood Donor Motivation and Recruitment," *Transfusion* 17, no. 2: 123–135 (1977); Oswalt, "A Review of the Experimental Control of Blood Donor Motivation," in *Research in Psychology and Medicine*, vol. II, edited by Osborne et al. (London: Academic, 1979). For a representative sample of readings from the literature on blood-donor motivation and recruitment see Selected Readings in Donor Motivation and Recruitment, vols. I and II (Washington, D.C.: American National Red Cross, 1969 and 1974).

2. During the 1972 fiscal year, a major study of the blood-services complex was performed for the National Heart and Lung Institute (now the National Heart, Lung, and Blood Institute) by the firm Booz Allen and Hamilton, Inc. The study had a very broad scope. It was an intense study conducted over a short time period, limiting its data-collection efforts. The analysis includes an estimate of about 9.4 million units of whole blood collected during 1971. Figures are given for units of blood collected by commercial firms that paid donors, but these do not include the then-frequent practice of payment to some donors by some hospitals and blood centers. An overview of the study and its conclusions are presented in the Summary Report of NHLI's Blood Resource Studies, DHEW publication (NIH) 73-416 (Washington, D.C.: U.S. Government Printing Office, 1972).

The 1973 Health Interview Survey, conducted by the National Center for Health Statistics (NCHS), included a small set of items about blood donation, concerned only with donation behavior during the previous 12 months. Limited to the civilian, noninstitutionalized population, this survey was subject to thorough statistical controls, and its respondents are an excellent representation of the general public. About 120,000 people living in about 41,000 households were in the sample. The survey analysis provided an estimate that a total of about 10.2 million blood donations were made by a total of about 6.5 million donors during a 12-month period. Because of underrepresentation of young and institutionalized people, NCHS believed its estimate to be somewhat lower than the actual collection level during 1973. About 8 percent of these donations were made for monetary payment. For some informative breakdowns of blood-donation data from the 1973 Health Interview Survey, see Blood Donor Characteristics and Types of Blood Donations, United States, 1973, Vital and Health Statistics: Series 10, Data from the National Health Survey, No. 106, DHEW publication (HRA) 76-1533 (Washington, D.C.: U.S. Government Printing Office, 1976). A slightly expanded set of questions were included in the 1978 Health Interview Survey, but tabulations have not been published as of August 1981.

Estimates of time series for several quantities relevant to blood collection have appeared in a study performed by an investment firm: K. S. Abramowitz and L. A. Sanders, Baxter Travenol Laboratories—Analysis of Blood Collection Equipment Industry and Implications for the Fenwal Division (New York: Sanford C. Bernstein and Company, 1978). Using data available from the major blood-collection organizations and some courage, the authors gave what appear to us to be reasonable but somewhat high estimates and forecasts for annual whole-blood donations from 1971 through 1982.

3. The research summarized in this chapter was performed under grant NIH-5-R01-HS01440, "Blood Donor Motivation and Recruitment," to the Operations Research Center of the Massachusetts Institute of Technology from the National Center for Health Services Research, H.R.A., U.S. Public Health Service. The primary project reports are Alvin W. Drake, Public Attitudes and Decision Processes With Regard to Blood Donation (1978) and Michael J. Caruso, Blood Donation Attitudes and Behavior (1978). Both may be purchased by writing to A. Drake, Room 35-212, MIT, Cambridge, Mass. 02139.

4. The general public, insurance companies, and high school survey activities were performed in the late spring and early summer of 1976. The frequent and former donor survey activity was performed in the fall of 1975. We are aware of no developments that suggest the character of the survey responses would have been significantly different if the activities reported on here had been repeated five years later.

5. Requests for replacement blood made to specific individuals are no longer a major factor in whole blood collection. The practice was far more common when many hospitals were forced to generate their own blood supplies. Although this is a powerful type of donor solicitation, it is not an effective way to generate a significant part of a community's blood supply.

6. Our estimate for the number of people in the United States medically

qualified to give blood was obtained by a method suggested by T. Miller et al. (Cost Analysis of Blood Banking Alternatives, NBS Technical Note 777, SD Catalog no. C13.46:777 [Washington, D.C.: U.S. Government Printing Office, 1973]) in which several detailed health statistics for factors that disqualify people from donating are applied to groupings by age and sex. The method probably underestimates the number of qualified donors. The report, which is much broader than its title implies, is summarized in Volume II of the ANRC Selected Readings referred to in note 1.

7. Blood Donor Characteristics and Types of Blood Donations United States, 1973 (listed in note 2).

8. Because the surveys were conducted at midyear, time intervals with half-years seemed appropriate. Use of the 3½-year interval here and in our later work with ex-donors allowed us to ask simply for respondents' estimates of the year in which they had made their most recent donations.

Chapter 8

1. It is interesting to compare the covers of the American and British paperback editions of Titmuss' *The Gift Relationship*. Both covers are illustrated with a gift-wrapped blood container. The American edition, however, used a plastic bag, while the British featured a glass bottle—presumably so that each would be better recognized in its home market.

2. Booz Allen Hamilton, Supply and Use of the Nation's Blood Resources, NHLI Blood Resources Studies, vol. I, 1972.

3. Council of Europe, The Production and Use of Cellular Blood Components for Transfusion (1976), p. 10, table II.

4. Much of this section is based on a study of blood banking done in 1974–1976 by Sapolsky and Finkelstein and reported as a review of Titmuss. See Harvey M. Sapolsky and Stan Finkelstein, "Blood Policy Revisited—A New Look at the 'Gift Relationship,' " *Public Interest*, Winter 1977, pp. 15–27.

5. *American Red Cross Blood Services Bulletin* 14, no. 20: 3 (1980).

6. The International Red Cross Conference held in Stockholm in 1948 passed a resolution establishing the principles of blood as a free gift. This position has been continually reaffirmed by The League of Red Cross Societies. See Z. S. Hantchef, "The Red Cross and New Developments in Blood Transfusion," *Bull. World Federation of Hemophilia*, no. 9 (June 1975).

7. 28th World Health Assembly, May 1975.

8. Council of Europe, Activities of the Subcommittee of Specialists on Blood Problems 1969–1974, Strasbourg, December 1974, p. 17. The statement is contained in the recommendations for 1973.

9. *Transfusion International*, no. 14 (September 1978), p. 8.

10. Z. S. Hantchef, The Red Cross and Some Aspects of the Trade in Blood, paper prepared for the Red Cross Blood Transfusion Expert Working Group, Teheran, October 1973, p. 3.

11. *Transfusion International,* no. 14 (September 1978), p. 8, reporting on symposium in *Vox Sanguinis* 34, no. 6 (1978).

12. U. Lassen et al., "A Sociological Study of Donor Recruitment," in *Medico-Social Documentation,* no. 32: 27 (1973).

13. *American Red Cross Blood Services Bulletin* 13, no. 21: 4 (1980).

14. *Medico-Social Documentation,* no. 18: 14 (1961).

15. Ken Auletta, *The Streets Were Paved With Gold* (New York: Random House, 1979), p. 149.

16. Dr. Morris of Australia at *Vox Sanguinis* symposium (see ref. 11).

17. Comments of G. A. Miterev in *Medico-Social Documentation,* no. 32: 23–24 (1973); L. K. Nikolaeva, D. I. Rafalson, and R. N. Shabashova, "Blood Donor Recruitment in the Soviet Union," part I, *Transfusion* 20, no. 3 (1980).

18. Miterev (ref. 17), p. 252. Miterev says "The gift of blood in the U.S.S.R. is a problem which has been solved; it is based on the fundamental principle: maximum aid to the sick, no danger whatever to the donor."

19. "Whole Blood and Red Cells," docket 75N–0316, U.S. Food and Drug Administration and 40 *Federal Register* 53040 (1975).

20. *American Red Cross Blood Services Bulletin* 13, no. 15: 6 (1980).

21. Z. S. Hantchef, "The Red Cross and New Developments," *Bull. World Federation of Hemophilia* (June 1975). Note also "The Red Cross and Blood Transfusion" map, League of Red Cross, Red Crescent, Red Lion and Sun Societies, January 1974.

22. Note for example Subcommittee of Specialists on Blood Problems, Council of Europe, The Production and Use of Cellular Blood Components for Transfusion, May 1975.

23. *Vox Sanguinis* 23: 63 (1972); *Transfusion International* no. 17 (May 1979): 5; Aaron Kellner and Carlos Ehrich, The Movement of Blood and Blood Products Across International Boundaries: The Cooperative and Non-Commercial Approach, unpublished.

24. *Transfusion International* no. 17 (May 1979): 4.

25. *Transfusion International* no. 17 (May 1979): 10–11 reports that 230,000 units of red cells were imported in 1978 under what is called the Euroblood program, an exchange between West Germany, Switzerland, and Belgium and the New York Blood Center and the American Red Cross. The blood is drawn in Europe under U.S. license and used primarily in New York City but also other areas in the United States.

26. Note also "Profiteering in Blood is Scored by WHO," *Washington Post,* May 17, 1975, and Mark Winiarski, "Blood Trade Drains Poor, Aids Rich," *National Catholic Reporter,* July 4, 1975.

27. *Vox Sanguinis* 23:63 (1972).

Index

Albumin, 64–65, 72–73
American Association of Blood Banks
  and American Blood Commission, 130, 131, 133
  on blood coverage, 133
  clearinghouse program of, 20, 53
  and cooperative efforts, 54–56, 130, 133
  and Council of Community Blood Centers, 53
  educational programs of, 23
  formation of, 50–52
  and government regulation, 133
  ideology of, 20–21, 46, 54
  membership of, 52–53, 57
  and Red Cross, 2, 46–47, 52–56, 141
  scientific orientation of, 52
  strains within, 57, 141
American Blood Commission
  community responsibility endorsed by, 132–133
  establishment of, 56, 130
  membership of, 130, 131
  National Blood Data Center under, 77
  on need for education, 81
  problems of, 132
  regionalization efforts by, 141, 142
American National Red Cross. *See* Red Cross
Antihemophilic factor, 64, 65
  and hepatitis, 66
  increased demand for, 72–73
  and profitability, 73–74
"Artificial blood," 2, 10, 135

Blood banking (whole blood)
  cross-national comparisons of, 114–116. *See also* Foreign nations
  and distribution, 7, 25–26
  financial considerations in, 27–28
  government regulation of, 62, 143
  interregional transfer in, 139
  stages in, 22
Blood centers, 6, 7
Blood Clearinghouse Program. *See* American Association of Blood Banks

Blood components, 9–11. *See also* Component therapy; Plasma
Blood credits, 5, 132
Blood donation. *See also* Donors; Plasma
  aftereffects of, 43–44, 70
  assumptions about, 76–77
  for components, 10
  eligibility for, 42–44, 85–86, 100
  incentives for, 1, 5–6, 23–24, 117–118, 139–140
  limiting factors in, 76, 81, 86, 104, 112, 113
  media treatment of, 1–2, 19, 23, 138–139
  nondonors' attitudes toward, 93, 95–96, 105–107
  opportunities for, 24, 83–85, 87, 90–94, 96, 100–103
  payment for. *See* Payment for blood donations
  process of, 4–5
  public attitudes toward, 89, 99–100, 103, 112–113, 137
  rate of, 4, 5, 22, 137
  reasons against, 90–94, 96
  reasons for, 97–100, 112
  voluntariness of, 117–118, 125
Blood needs, 12, 22, 97, 137
  personal closeness to, 81–83
Blood plasma. *See* Plasma
Blood quality
  and donor-recipient incompatibility, 42
  hepatitis as threat to, 29, 30–32, 40, 45. *See also* Hepatitis
  and infectious diseases, 41
  and red-blood-cell potency, 41–42
"Boston Agreement," 54, 55

Center for Disease Control, 31
Clotting proteins, 65–66, 72–73
Cohn fractionation, 61, 63, 64
Commercial collecting agencies. *See also* Plasma industry
  attacks on, 62–63
  attitudes toward, 107–108

Commercial collecting agencies (cont.)
  decline of, 63, 122, 135
  demand for, 6–7, 127–128
  and foreign countries, 122, 136
  and hepatitis risk, 33, 128
  vs. nonprofit collection, 114–115, 122, 125, 127–128, 136
Committee on Commonality in Blood Bank Automation, 42
Component therapy
  and hepatitis risk, 39–40
  and whole-blood supply, 9–10, 12
Council of Community Blood Centers, 53, 57, 130, 132, 133, 141
Council of Europe, Public Health Committee of, 117
CR. See Ideologies
CR-MC. See Ideologies
Crossmatching, 26, 28. See also Transfusion
CR-SG. See Ideologies

Diagnostic reagents, 66, 67
Donor groups, 16–17
Donors, distribution of
  by age, 87–88
  by number of donations, 88–89
  by sex, 87–88

Eligibility to donate blood
  and ex-donors, 100
  perceptions of, 85–86

Foreign nations. See also Great Britain
  blood banking in, 120–121
  donation-payment policies in, 69, 117–120, 125
  ideologies in, 124
  and plasma banking, 67–74, 121–124, 136

Gamma globulins. See Immune proteins
Gift Relationship, The (Titmuss), 3, 56, 62, 114–115, 124
Great Britain, 114–116, 120

Health, Education and Welfare, Department of, 63, 129
Health and Scientific Research Subcommittee (U.S. Senate), 2–3
Hepatitis
  characteristics of, 29–30
  posttransfusion, 3, 30–41, 45, 66, 115–116, 119, 128, 134–136
  research on, 134
  testing for, 25, 134
High schools, blood donation at, 89, 90, 105–107

Ideologies, blood-collection
  of American Association of Blood Banks, 20, 21, 46, 54, 80
  vs. actual practices, 18–20, 24
  in blood-donation study, 80, 97–99, 107–112
  CR (community responsibility), 13–14, 110–112
  CR-MC, 15–16, 124
  CR-SG, 16, 24, 98, 124
  and donors' reasons, 99, 108–109, 112, 140
  in foreign countries, 124
  IR (individual responsibility), 13–14, 110–112, 124
  IR-MC, 16–17, 22, 24, 97–99
  IR-SG, 17–18
  and jurisdictional variations, 18
  MC (market commodity), 14–15
  questions determining, 13–15
  and Red Cross, 21, 46, 53–54, 80
  SG (special gift), 14–15
Immune proteins, 65
International Federation of Blood Donor Associations, 117
International Society of Blood Transfusion, 117
Interregional sharing of blood supply, 139
IR. See Ideologies
IR-MC. See Ideologies
IR-SG. See Ideologies

Joint Blood Council, 55
Journey (R. and S. Massie), 3

League of Red Cross Societies, 116

MC. See Ideologies

National Blood Data Center, 77, 130
National Blood Policy
  and American Blood Commission, 130
  and use of commercial blood, 63
  goals of, 129
  Senate hearings on, 2–3

Index

National Center for Health Services Research, 77
National Health Interview Survey (1978), 89
National Heart and Lung Institute, 115
National Transfusion Hepatitis Study, 31, 33
Nonprofit organizations. *See* American Association of Blood Banks; Red Cross

Payment for blood donations. *See also* Commercial collecting agencies
  attitudes toward, 95, 96, 107, 108–109, 111, 112, 128–129
  expense of, 28
  extent of, 7, 138
  and hepatitis, 32–36, 115–116
  and plasma industry, 9, 66–67, 70
Pharmaceutical sector. *See also* Plasma industry
  and blood plasma, 7–9
  and component therapy, 10
Plasma. *See also* Plasmapheresis
  derivatives from, 8, 63–66, 72–73
  and disease, 136
  sources of, 67
Plasma industry, 60–63, 66–75. *See also* Pharmaceutical sector
  collection for, 8–9, 66–70, 122, 136
  development of, 60–63
  and Food and Drug Administration, 136
  in foreign countries, 72, 121–123, 136
  foreign trade in, 67–74, 123–124
  fractionation facilities of, 71–75
  future of, 72, 74–75
  profitability of, 73–74, 136–137
Plasmapheresis
  aftereffects of, 70
  and ideology, 13
  new techniques for, 74, 137
  process of, 8–9
  and voluntary donation, 74
  and whole-blood collection, 8, 67, 121–122, 135–137
Processing, of collected blood, 25
Profit-making organizations. *See* Commercial collecting agencies; Plasma industry

Recruitment. *See* Solicitation of donors
Red Cross, American National
  and American Association of Blood Banks, 2, 46–47, 54–56, 141
  and American Blood Commission, 130–133
  blood banking started by, 46, 48–52
  and Blood Clearinghouse Program, 55, 132
  on blood credits, 132–133
  collection programs of, 6
  and collection shortfalls, 127, 128
  and cooperative efforts, 54–56, 130, 133
  and Council of Community Blood Centers, 53
  distribution management by, 25–26
  and donation payment, 119
  educational programs of, 23
  financing under, 59
  functions of, 47–48
  and ideology, 21, 46, 53–54
  national-vs.-local friction in, 49
  organization of, 49, 57, 58
  plasma fractionation by, 59, 75
  strains within, 49, 57–59, 141
  and threat of government regulation, 133
Red Cross, foreign
  blood-banking role of, 120, 121
  and payment for donation, 116, 118
Regionalization, 134, 140–143

Schweicker, Sen. Richard, 3
SG. *See* Ideologies
Solicitation of donors, 22–25
  and ex-donors, 100, 102–103
  extent of, 83–85
  intense environments for, 103–104
  and nondonors' reasons, 90–94, 96

Transfusions
  conditions requiring, 11–12
  consent for, 42
  costs of, 2–3
  misutilization in, 27
  quality of, 45
  recipients of, 11

World Federation of Hemophilia, 117
World Health Organization, 116–117